THE
CLEANSING
Power of Yoga

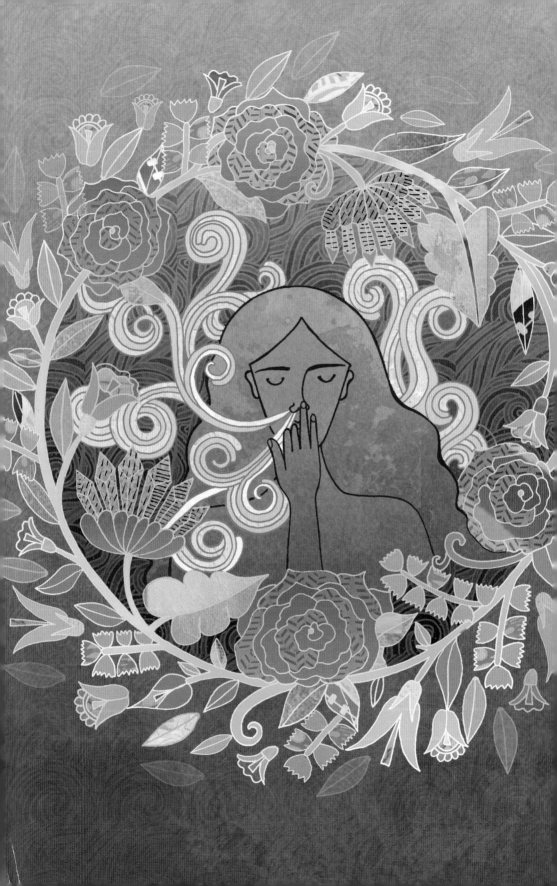

THE
CLEANSING
Power of Yoga

Kriyas and other holistic detox
techniques for health and wellbeing

Swami Saradananda

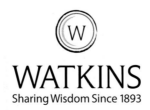

WATKINS
Sharing Wisdom Since 1893

The Cleansing Power of Yoga
Swami Saradananda

First published in the UK and USA in 2018 by
**Watkins, an imprint of Watkins Media
Limited**
Unit 11, Shepperton House,
83–93 Shepperton Road
London N1 3DF

enquiries@watkinspublishing.com

ISBN: 978-1-78678-167-3
10 9 8 7 6 5 4 3 2 1
Typeset in Agenda
Colour reproduction by XY Digital
Printed in China

Commissioning Editor: Kelly Thompson
Managing Editor: Daniel Hurst
Editor: Susannah Marriott
Head of Design: Georgina Hewitt
Production: Uzma Taj
Commissioned photography: Christina Wilson
Commissioned artwork: Hannah Davies

A CIP record for this book is available from the
British Library

Note/Disclaimer: The material contained in
this book is set out in good faith for general
guidance and no liability can be accepted for
any loss, injury or expense incurred in relying
on the information given. In particular this
book is not intended to replace expert medical
or psychiatric advice. This book is for
informational purposes only and is for your
own personal use and guidance. It is not
intended to diagnose, treat or act as a
substitute for professional medical advice.
The author is not a medical practitioner nor
a counsellor, and professional advice should
be sought if desired before embarking on any
health-related programme.

Notes: Abbreviations used throughout this
book: CE Common Era (the equivalent of AD)
BCE Before Common Era (the equivalent of BC)
b. born, d. died

www.watkinspublishing.com

DEDICATION

I dedicate this book to my teachers as well as to my students, many of whom have taught and inspired me.

'apyayantu mamangani vak pranas caksuh srotram
atho balam indriyani ca sarvani'

'May my limbs, speech, prana, sight, hearing, strength and all my senses, gain in vigour'

'OM Shanti Shanti Shanti'

'OM Peace Peace Peace'

Shanti manta, found in both Kena and Chandogya Upanishads

'By whom is the mind commanded and directed to go towards its objects? Who causes the prana to move? By whose will do people utter speech? What power directs the eye and the ear?

It is the ear of the ear, the mind of the mind, the speech of the speech, the prana of the prana, the eye of the eye. The wise, freed (from the pull of the senses and from false notions), renounce this world and become immortal.'

Kena Upanishad, 1.1-2

CONTENTS

INTRODUCTION

A yogic lifestyle is one of simple living and positive thinking. It goes beyond the purely postural forms that most people know as yoga, and encompasses the cleansing practices known as *kriyas* in Sanskrit, which offer a natural way to eliminate any tension, physical impurities and energetic blockages that can inhibit your enjoyment of radiant good health. In this book I present a variety of these techniques designed to purify body and mind.

Although this is a book about yoga, most of the exercises it contains are not designed to increase your strength or flexibility. They may well be unlike any yoga practices you are used to – and yet when you start performing these cleansing rituals regularly you may well notice that you feel stronger and more flexible. As your body becomes purified, you will notice your health improving. As your mind becomes purified, you will find yourself feeling increasingly clear, friendly and cheerful. You will begin to realize that happiness comes not from the external objects and circumstances that bring a little transient pleasure, but from within your own being. Your body, thoughts and emotions will become vibrant reflections of your inner self.

Yoga cleansing has much to offer us in the 21st century. It is helpful if you find it difficult to reduce tension, eat properly, get a good night's sleep or enough rest, if you constantly feel stressed or try to force yourself beyond your limits. It is effective if you live in a city or town, work with other people, go to restaurants and shops or travel on public transport, when it is almost impossible not to pick up other people's ailments and negative energies. You may worry that your food is adulterated with empty calories, processed sugars and unhealthy additives, that your water is not clean and your environment contaminated with airborne toxins, noise and light pollution. This all contributes to increased stress levels that can weaken your body. If you do not feel at ease or comfortable in your skin, dis-ease may follow, and then even a regular yoga-posture practice can fail to bring about the inner joyfulness that yoga promises.

Kriyas actively counter this by ridding your body of accumulated impurities and strengthening the subtle energy channels that are the interface between your physical being and thought processes. The integration that results can be valuable in preventing and healing a range of chronic disorders. Regular practice also helps to remove many of the obstacles that prevent you from engaging positively with the world around you.

It takes very little time to practise kriyas – it's easy, for example, to build them into your morning routine. They are effective whether or not you already practise yoga postures or observe other yoga teachings. However, when you incorporate cleansing exercises into a regular routine of yoga postures and also combine them with a diet based around whole plant foods, they can be immensely valuable in helping you to experience a positive state of glowing, joyful wellbeing that is much more than the simple negation of disease.

Alongside the feeling of physical purity that comes with regular yoga cleansing, mental clarity develops and a lifting of the cloud that hides the immensity and luminosity of your true self; your connection to others blossoms and you start to reflect the wonder of life more completely in all your relationships. As you begin to include some of the cleansing practices in this book into your daily routine, I hope you will be amazed at their positive effects.

Swami Saradananda

"The expression of the spirit increases in proportion to the development of the body and mind in which it is encased"
Swami Vishnu-devananda,
Complete Illustrated Book of Yoga

WOULD YOU BENEFIT FROM YOGA CLEANSING?

If you answer yes to any of the following questions you will find techniques in the book to help you:

- Would you like to improve your general health and wellbeing?
- Do you need to reduce physical stress and ease anxiety?
- Do you lack focus or concentration?
- Would you like to clear your mind, body and environment of clutter?
- Do you notice a thick coating on your tongue when you wake in the morning?
- Do you tire more easily than you used to or increasingly lack stamina?
- Are you aware of a lack of healthy motivation in your life?
- Would you like to increase your energy levels?
- Are you keen to improve your quality of sleep?
- Do you often catch colds or suffer recurrent headaches?
- Do you regularly consume and crave junk foods, sugar and caffeinated drinks?
- Are you are plagued by feelings of heaviness or bloating?
- Do you suffer from chronic constipation or other digestive problems?
- Would you like to strengthen your immune system?
- Do you have difficulty in setting yourself healthy boundaries?
- Are you looking to ease tensions in your relationships?
- Would you like to feel more joy and enthusiasm for life in general?

THE ROOTS OF YOGA CLEANSING

This book aims to put the teachings of yoga, ancient and modern, on purifying body and mind – *shaucha* in Sanskrit – into everyday language, and to inspire you with simple ways to integrate them into your life. The detoxification, or detox, process helps to rid the body of accumulated physical "contaminants" and the mind and emotions of "impurities" that may have undesirable effects on your health and wellbeing. Many lifestyle programmes offer similar detox strategies, from fasting to avoiding specific foods and cleansing the organs of elimination – but none go so deeply into purification on all levels as the yoga tradition, which encourages you to see your body as the vehicle or temple of your soul.

The ancient yoga sage Patanjali first speaks of shaucha, physical and mental purification, in the classic text known as the *Yoga Sutra*, in which the precepts of this ancient science were compiled between 200 BCE and 400 CE. Here he presents an eight-limbed path for living joyously and reaching your greatest potential. Of all the paths of yoga, Patanjali's psychological approach is the most scientific and easily applied to a modern lifestyle. Never has the human mind been so thoroughly analysed or the process of eliminating human frailties so succinctly presented. Although ancient in origin, the eight principles he sets out are powerful tools to help alleviate many stresses of modern life (see opposite).

To find the actual techniques to detoxify mind and body, we need to consult the hatha yoga texts. Composed in the medieval period, these offer a guide to cleansing mind and body energetically (see pages 18–19) as well as physically. The mid-15th century *Hatha Yoga Pradipika* sets out the *shad-kriyas* or six cleansing techniques (see page 15), while the most practical and systematic text *Gheranda Samhita*, composed in the late 17th century, offers 21 different kriyas. Twentieth-century Indian yogis, including Dhirendra Brahmachari and Swami Satyananda, elaborated on traditional practices, making them more widely known.

PATANJALI'S EIGHT-LIMBED PATH OF PURIFICATION

Patanjali's *Yoga Sutra* remains the standard guide for a "pure" yoga lifestyle. By following its advice you will gain a great deal of wisdom and a more peaceful outlook – even if you don't become fully enlightened! Patanjali acknowledges that each of us possesses vast mental and psychic resources, many of which lie virtually untapped below the surface of the conscious mind. In the *Yoga Sutra* he prescribes a process of self-enquiry to help you access these super-powers and bring about personal change. It is based on a firm foundation of ethics, morals, posture and breath control plus ways to reign in your senses from their focus on external objects. Only when your foundation is firm, he teaches, can you build a successful superstructure of concentration and meditation. Patanjali's yoga comprises eight (*ashta* in Sanskrit) branches or parts (*anga*) that make body and mind more pure, flexible and strong:

1 **Yamas:** guidance on what not to do, from avoiding violence to being truthful (see pages 12–13). These are the boundaries and ethical guidelines that govern both your yoga practice and the way you interact with other people. The principles of yama help you to simplify your life so you can be at peace with yourself and the world beyond you.
2 **Niyamas:** guidance on what to do, from leading a simple life to self-study (see page 13). These principles are about self-discipline and govern your attitudes to and relationship with yourself. Following the niyamas gives you a positive way to take responsibility for your actions.
3 **Asana:** finding a "steady seat", or being able to remain in a position that is relaxed, firm and comfortable. The regular practice of yoga postures (*asanas* in Sanskrit) prepares both your body and mind for meditation.
4 **Pranayama:** controlling and elongating your subtle energy, *prana*, beginning with the physical breath.
5 **Pratyahara:** drawing your mental energy inward and shutting off the outward movement of your senses by using sense-withdrawal techniques. These turn the direction of your flow of consciousness inward, helping to prepare your mind for meditation.
6 **Dharana:** concentration.
7 **Dhyana:** meditation; the experience of inner peace.
8 **Samadhi:** enlightenment, or the super-conscious state in which you experience the unity of all things and become absorbed in the Absolute.

WHY CLEANSING STARTS WITH ETHICS

Patanjali doesn't advise you to start a yoga practice by performing yoga postures or by sitting to meditate. Instead, he begins with the ethical teachings known in Sanskrit as the *yamas* and *niyamas*. Why do the first steps on the path of yoga involve good conduct? Because it is essential that you purify your motives as well as your body and mind when you start to practise yoga.

It is believed that most people use between five and ten percent of their mental potential. Starting a yoga practice tends to enhance many latent capacities in your personality, and as these develop, your mind becomes more powerful. Unless you have spiritual integrity and discipline, such new-found powers of mind can be distracting, affecting you and others in negative ways. The ancient *rishis*, or yoga sages, were aware of the natural tendency for strong minds to control weaker minds. Realizing that power corrupts, they ensured the first steps on the path of yoga – the yamas and niyamas – purified mind, body and motives, forming a sound foundation for a balanced practice.

Yoga practice also tends to speed up your karma (the consequences of past actions), potentially accelerating your spiritual progress and intensifying the need for ethical behaviour. As you live with and practise yoga ethics and morals, you will find your behaviour and thoughts start to change, becoming purer and leading you in more positive directions. The yamas and niyamas are not harsh rules, but rather a description of human potential. They offer you a way to start living with deeper integrity and joy.

THE YAMAS

Personal restraints known as yamas help you to regulate the way in which you relate to the world outside yourself and to other people. The reverence you bring to daily living reinforces your sense of the sacredness of all life. It is no coincidence that Gandhi worked so hard at sanitation efforts in both South Africa and India.

Ahimsa: non-violence, or refraining from doing injury. Ahimsa is the ultimate weapon of a strong person. By practising being kind and compassionate in your actions, words and thoughts you purify any aggression in your nature.

Satya: truthfulness, refraining from lying. Truthfulness and ahimsa always go together. Attempting to tune into truth in the greatest sense is not always easy, but searching for it cleanses your mind and inner resolve.

Asteya: non-stealing. This means refraining from misappropriation and jealousy; it is all about not wanting what is not rightfully yours.

Aparigraha: non-greediness. A form of non-possessiveness, this covers everything from refusing bribes to not being overly grasping. It may be seen as freeing yourself from the rigidity of society's dictates, or living without surplus possessions, and encourages you to discern the difference between what you need and what you want.

Brahmacharya: not allowing your mind to dwell on the sensory. This yama is about self-control and your ability to resist the outward (and downward) pull of sensuality. Brahmacharya transforms physical energy (*ojas*) into spiritual brilliance (*tejas*).

THE NIYAMAS
These five principles are the spiritual laws to better control your instincts and emotions and find the most positive ways to relate to yourself. The first of the niyamas, shaucha (purification on all levels) is the most relevant to this book. Purifying body and mind helps you find balance and is a pre-condition for experiencing everything else yoga can offer.

Shaucha: internal and external cleanliness. By observing shaucha you create a pure environment for a yoga practice while purging heart and mind of unhealthy attachments or obsessions. It includes the physical cleanliness that results from regularly cleansing the body, maintaining an orderly home, eating healthy food and drinking clean water. But it also relates to mental clarity and speaking without using emotionally charged language.

Santosha: contentment. This niyama is all about being happy with who you are while cultivating inner peace and spiritual growth.

Tapas: austerity or voluntary simplicity. Just by trying to live a simpler life, you "burn off" physical, mental and emotional impurities.

Svadhyaya: self-study. This niyama is not about an intellectual gathering of information, but attempting to better understand your inner nature.

Ishvara-pranidhana: letting go of the idea that you are separate from the rest of nature. As this quality develops you surrender to a higher power, however you understand it.

WHAT ARE KRIYA CLEANSING EXERCISES?

Whether you already practise yoga, are thinking of taking it up, or would simply like more clarity in your life, cleansing exercises can help you achieve your goals, reduce any resistance you might have to positive change and give you a fresh outlook. The practices mentioned in this book are tools that can help you both on and off the yoga mat or meditation cushion. They are designed to begin a cleansing process that will enhance every aspect of your life.

Most traditional yoga systems and many schools of modern postural yoga encompass more than just the physical poses (asanas). They also advocate breathing exercises (pranayama), energetic seals (mudras), bodily locks (bandhas), meditations (focusing on the chakras) and cleansing techniques (kriyas). All these practices are designed to cleanse and strengthen the meridians or energetic passageways referred to as *nadis* by yoga practitioners through which the subtle energy or life-force known as *prana* travels (see pages 18–19). They work to centralize prana in the energy channels and raise your "vibratory level", which makes your mind and body more sensitive and intuitive. Practising kriyas regularly helps to increase your vibratory level in as short a time as possible, awakening your dormant potential, known as *kundalini*, and transforming it from static energy into a dynamic state.

To understand the importance of cleansing exercises, it can be helpful to use an electrical metaphor. Some substances, such as copper, are good conductors of electricity, but if they become corrupted with impurities, the conductivity is reduced. Similarly, if your physical and energetic bodies (see pages 16–17) contain impurities, there is greater resistance to the healthy flow of energy. By steadily practising cleansing exercises, you remove any impurities and restore conductivity.

It's easy to start adding one or two kriyas to your daily routine. When they become habitual, just add in one or two more. In fact you're probably doing some of the kriyas already simply by washing your hands and showering regularly. An easy extension would be to get into the habit of washing your hands whenever you return from a public place, then shake them vigorously for 10–20 seconds.

Don't feel pressured to do too much yoga cleansing at once or to practise too deeply or too fast: adding to your repertoire of cleansing exercises slowly and staying within your personal capacity is the most effective way to purify and strength your nadi energy channels. Practising more intensively doesn't necessarily bring better results.

THE SIX CLEANSING ACTIONS OF YOGA: SHAD-KRIYA

According to the *Hatha Yoga Pradipika*, there are six classical yoga cleansing acts that purify the body: they work on the upper digestive tract (Dhauti, see page 106), colon (Basti, see page 110), nasal passages (Neti, see page 74), the eyes and front of the body (Tratak, see page 36), the abdomen (Nauli, see page 108) and the respiratory organs (Kapalabhati , see page 76). All six acts are held in high esteem by the great yogis.

In addition, yoga philosophy recommends energetic "seals" known as mudras that direct prana for a cleansing effect, as well as certain bandhas or bodily "locks" that secure prana into positive channels, and you will find examples throughout the book.

BEST TIME TO PRACTISE

The most effective times to practise cleansing exercises are at dawn and dusk when the atmosphere is charged with a special spiritual force. It is also best to practise before eating. Modern lifestyles often make it difficult to practise at sunrise and sunset, so you might like to choose a time to do cleansing exercises when you are not involved in everyday activities and your mind is able to focus on the practice at hand.

Many people find it convenient to practise kriyas in the morning, perhaps on waking; your mind is still in a "pure" state at this time and hasn't yet become involved in the work of the day. Or you might like to practise in the evening, after putting aside the cares of the day, when you can devote some quiet time to cleansing your inner environment.

Alternatively, practising later at night can be an effective way of cleansing your mind before you go to bed. If you can calm and purify your mind by doing kriyas, you may find that you fall into deep sleep more quickly, rest more effectively and wake up in the morning feeling really energized.

Every day is a good day to cleanse. But the change of seasons – when summer becomes autumn and winter becomes spring – are considered the best times for a more intense cleanse. These are the most advantageous periods for sloughing off any toxins you may have accumulated over the previous few months.

Often people say they would like to develop a cleansing practice, but don't have the time. Whenever that thought comes to mind, remind yourself that developing a regular cleansing routine can help you to work more efficiently, feel calmer and more centred, and perhaps even reduce your need for sleep, giving you more useful hours in the day.

CLEANSING THE THREE BODIES

In order to understand more about how the cleansing techniques in this book work and can help in your daily life, it's useful to gain a little understanding of yoga philosophy and the model it postulates of three bodies: the physical body, astral body and causal body. Each is more subtle and less easy to understand than the previous one.

YOUR PHYSICAL BODY

The most concrete of the three bodies is the one you are most familiar with. This is your physical body, thought by yogis to be made up of food and to go back into the food cycle when it dies. You can purify your physical body by practising:

• Yoga postures (asanas).

• These cleansing exercises (kriyas) in particular: Neti (see page 74), Nauli (see page 108), Dhauti (see page 106), Basti (see page 110), Kapalabhati (see page 76), Tratak (see page 36).

• A "pure" diet (see pages 98–99) and occasional fasting (see pages 100–101).

YOUR ASTRAL BODY

Like most people interested in yoga, you probably realize that greater dimensions to life lie beyond the "reality" of the physical body. The astral, or subtle, body is the second body. It is the one believed to reincarnate, taking a new physical body at birth. Death is defined as the total separation of the astral and physical bodies. Your astral body contains your personality and thoughts, likes and dislikes – all your qualities and emotions that are non-physical. To understand the concept, think about how emotions like love or fear affect your body – your heart or bowels, for example – even though the emotions are not physical. While they strongly affect your physical body, emotions have their seat in your astral body – like your mind, intellect and the subtle energy yogis call *prana*. Your astral body has three "sheaths" or layers, known as *koshas* in Sanskrit.

The **first layer** or vital sheath, *pranamaya kosha*, contains your subtle energy, or life-force, as well as the channels through which it flows (nadis) and the centres (chakras) that receive and transmit this energy (see page 18). This "etheric double" sheath lies closest to your physical body, its energy flowing through and interpenetrating it as water fills a sponge. This is the layer of the body at which you experience sensations like hunger, thirst, heat and cold. You can purify this layer of your astral body by practising:

• Pranayama breath-control techniques.

- Speaking in a "pure" way: by not gossiping and saying what you mean (see page 60).
- Voluntary silence, or Mouna (see page 61).
- Chakra-cleansing techniques and chakra meditation.
- Mantra repetition.

The **second layer** of the astral body, the *manomaya kosha*, is the intellectual layer, where you experience emotions from anger to excitement. The senses (smell, taste, sight, touch and hearing) are based here, as is your automatic mind, with its conscious, subconscious and instinctive portions. This layer gets clogged by psychological and sensory distractions, attachments to past experiences, bondage to the demands of the body and anticipation of future events. You can purify this layer of the body by practising:
- Yoga postures (asanas), with relaxed breathing to calm your mind and emotions.
- Pranayama breath-control techniques.
- Chanting or singing.
- Selfless deeds, or Karma Yoga (see pages 148–9).
- Pratyahara, withdrawing from the senses (see page 11).
- Mindfulness and meditation.

The **third layer** of the astral body, the *vijnanamaya kosha*, is the intellectual layer, where you have doubts, debate with yourself and make decisions. It comprises your intellect (*buddhi*) and sense of unique individuality (*ahamkara*): your ego or who you perceive yourself to be. This separates you from identifying with universal consciousness. If you are interested in inner or spiritual work, you can purify your intellect and ego by practising:
- Selfless deeds, or Karma Yoga (see pages 148–9).
- Positive thinking and meditation.
- Focused inquiry and on-going study.

YOUR CAUSAL BODY

Yoga philosophy teaches that you also have a "causal" or seed body where your karma (consequences of past actions) and subtle impressions from this and past lives are stored. It also contains the seed that determines your talents and aptitudes, emotional make-up and physical appearance. Your causal body has one layer, the bliss sheath or *anandamaya kosha*, where you experience joy. You can purify your causal body by practising:
- Meditation.
- Selfless deeds, or Karma Yoga (see pages 148–9).

PURIFYING PRANA,
YOUR VITAL ENERGY

There is a subtle energy that surrounds and energizes the physical body that yogis refer to using the Sanskrit word *prana*. Although it flows through and animates your physical body, it is not a physical energy, nor is it made up of physical elements – prana is quite different from the electrical currents that move through your nervous system.

Prana flows through subtle channels known as *nadis* in the pranamaya kosha layer of your astral body (see page 16). It is estimated that approximately 72,000 nadis, referred to as "meridians" in acupuncture, make up the subtle wiring system of your astral body. Three nadis are of particular interest to yoga practitioners and so to those interested in yoga cleansing: *ida*, which flows to the left of your spine, *pingala* which flows to the right and the *sushumna* channel in the centre, approximating the spine.

A useful way to understand the concept is to visualize the nadis as roads on a highway system that allow traffic (your prana) to move around. A junction where two or more roads meet is more likely to become blocked than a straight, uninterrupted stretch of highway. And the more roads there are coming together, the more likelihood that a traffic jam will develop.

Any place where major nadis cross is referred to as a *chakra*, a junction of vibrant energy. Many smaller chakras are used as acupuncture points. Points where multiple nadis cross are known as minor or major chakras. The seven major chakras are located along the sushumna nadi. Each one acts as an organizational centre, receiving, assimilating and expressing energy, and is strongly connected to a different sense, type of emotion and quality of mind and body (see opposite). Each one works on a different precious piece of the puzzle of human consciousness. This makes it especially important to keep the chakra energy junctions clear so that prana can flow unimpeded throughout the nadi system. Yogis have developed various cleansing exercises to open and cleanse the nadis and chakras – for vibrant good health we need an unimpeded flow of prana throughout the body.

CLEANSING THE SEVEN MAJOR CHAKRAS

Acting as the interface between your physical body and its etheric double, the pranamaya kosha, chakras can be thought of as multi-dimensional balls of radiant energy. As each chakra vibrates at a different rate, its cleansing takes a different form.

1 Root (*muladhara*) chakra at the base of your body is connected with grounding and security and is the seat of a vast potential energy known as kundalini. It is associated with your sense of smell.

Purify with: the earth element, including eating grounding plant foods and eating when hungry rather than to fill emotional needs. Also by releasing fear and negative habits and behaviour patterns.

2 Sacral (*swadhisthana*) chakra around the middle of your lower back embodies creative energy and is the seat of your sexuality, plans and desire. It is associated with your sense of taste.

Purify with: the water element, including water-only fasts, sweating in a sauna or steam room, taking warm baths with mineral salts. Also by letting go of guilt and shame.

3 Solar plexus (*manipura*) chakra is your body's power centre and site of your digestive fire and willpower. It is associated with your sense of sight.

Purify with: yoga twisting poses, active (fiery) activities such as running or dancing, sharing food with friends. Also by releasing disempowering thoughts and detaching from anger.

4 Heart (*anahata*) chakra is connected with compassion and love. It is associated with your sense of touch.

Purify with: the air element, including deep breathing and pranayama breath-control techniques. Also by forgiving yourself and those you feel have injured you, learning from mistakes and moving on, grieving fully then letting go.

5 Throat (*vishuddha*) chakra is your centre of communication and creative flow. It is associated with your sense of hearing.

Purify with: sound and mantra repetition. Also by giving thanks before meals and expressing gratitude for life's blessings, speaking the truth, avoiding "toxic" language and making sure your words, thoughts and deeds are cohesive and authentic.

6 Brow (*ajna*) chakra, commonly referred to as the "third eye", is the seat of intuition, imagination and your purpose in life.

Purify with: positive thoughts and prayer. Also by avoiding violent films and TV shows.

7 Crown (*sahasrara*) chakra at the crown of your head is your connection to infinite potential.

Purify with: sunlight, meditation and communion with a higher consciousness.

AYURVEDIC CONSTITUTIONS

Cleansing techniques are found in many therapeutic approaches, such as reflexology and kinesiology, but in order to better understand how yogic cleansing works, it is helpful to have a basic knowledge of how Ayurveda, the best known traditional healing system of India, perceives the body and mind. Much of the basic philosophy is shared with yoga, and there is a frequent overlap of practices, though whereas yoga is a self-practice method, Ayurveda is a medical system in which treatments such as medicine and massage are prescribed and administered by a doctor or therapist.

Ayurveda recognizes three basic types of physical and mental make-up. These three constitutions, known as *doshas*, are composed of three energetic types: *vata*, *pitta* and *kapha*. Ayurvedic medicine places great emphasis on keeping them in balance. Many factors, internal and external, can disturb the balance of one or more of the doshas, including emotional and physical stress, eating the wrong diet for your body type, the seasons and weather, work, family and relationships. Cleansing yoga practices are a powerful way to help counteract many negative influences on your constitution and can play an important part in maintaining a healthy balance of the three doshas within your body, mind and consciousness.

THE THREE ENERGIES IN BALANCE

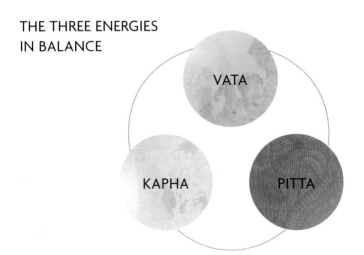

Yoga cleansing keeps the three energies in balance for optimal physical and emotional health.

KAPHA

This is the basic energy that forms the structure of your body and provides the foundation for the other doshas. Kapha is made up of the elements water (liquid matter) and earth (solid matter) and it is cold, moist and white in nature. It is stable and tends to move little.

When kapha is excessive, you may feel stuck in life, crave sweets, feel heavy and suffer from swelling of the body and general congestion. Respiratory and skin problems are said to result from kapha imbalance. Other symptoms may include bouts of depression, lethargy, passivity, weight gain, asthma and water retention.

Cleanse and rebalance with: active kriyas, such as Agni Sara and Kapalabhati (see page 76). In addition to these more vigorous cleanses, engage in gentle movement by practising yoga postures or talking regular walks.

VATA

The energy of movement, vata is made up of the elements air (matter in gaseous form) and ether (space). It is constantly moving, expansive in nature, easily changeable, irregular, cold and icy blue in colour.

When vata is excessive, your body tends to suffer from dryness, roughness, stiffness, joint pain, and brittle bones and teeth. You may have trouble focusing or committing to things. Joint problems and disorders relating to the nervous system are said to indicate an imbalance of vata energy.

Cleanse and rebalance with: exercises involving oils such as Oil Pulling (see page 96) – these tend to pacify and calm the excessive movement of the air element in space.

PITTA

The energy of digestion, assimilation and metabolism is considered to be pitta. It consists of the fire element and is hot, dry and bright red. Pitta generates heat in your body and regulates body temperature.

When pitta is excessive, you may get angry, suffer from high blood pressure or burning sensations, sweat too much and crave spicy food. Eczema, blotchy red skin, rashes, hives and irritability are said to be a result of pitta imbalance, as are digestive problems.

Cleanse and rebalance with: Liver Cleanse (see pages 102–103) . Also reduce your intake of coffee, tea and other stimulants in your diet.

THE FIVE CLEANSING ACTIONS OF AYURVEDA: PANCHA KARMA

The Sanskrit term *pancha karma* is often mistakenly used as a general term for Ayurvedic treatment. It actually refers to five (*pancha*) specific and very powerful detoxification techniques, which it is useful to know about (see below). Before undergoing these five *karmas* (actions), the patient consumes large amounts of ghee (clarified butter) and undergoes svedhana (sweat therapy or a steam bath) and abhyanga (oil massage). Of these five deep-cleansing techniques, you will find two self-practice exercises in the book: the nasal oil cleanse Nasya (see page 84) and the sweating treatment Svedhana (see pages 116–17). The other three treatments should only be undertaken under the care of a qualified Ayurvedic doctor or therapist.

PANCHA KARMA TREATMENT

A course of pancha karma supervised by an Ayurvedic practitioner includes the following treatments. After the course has been completed, rejuvenating herbs (*rasayana*) are prescribed.

1 Excess kapha is eliminated: using induced medical vomiting (*Vamana*).
2 This is followed by the nasal oil-cleansing technique Nasya (see page 116–17) to reduce kapha further.
3 Excess pitta is reduced by purging techniques (*Virechana*), including herbs taken orally to induce bowel elimination.

4 This is followed by detoxification of the blood (*Rakta Mokshana*) to reduce pitta further.

5 Finally, excess vata is eliminated, either using an oil enema (*Anuvasana*) or decoction enema (*Nirooha*), for which Basti (see page 110) may be substituted.

"Like an unbaked clay pot when put in water, the body is always decaying. Bake it with the fire of yoga and make it pure." Gheranda Samhita, 1, 8

CLARIFYING YOUR SENSES AND MIND

Practising the yoga cleansing exercises in this book will in turn help you enhance your sense-withdrawal techniques (pratyahara), the fifth stage in Patanjali's path toward a yoga lifestyle (see pages 10–11). When you shut off the outward movement of the senses you turn your flow of consciousness inward, making your mind more pure and preparing you for meditation.

Normally your knowledge of the world is fed by the reports your mind receives from your senses: sight, hearing, taste, touch and smell. In yoga philosophy, these are referred to as the *jnana indriyas*, or faculties of knowledge. Some people might think of the senses as passive receptors of impressions – you hear something because the sound comes into your ear. But in yoga tradition, the senses are perceived to actively move out into the world through the portals of your eyes, ears, nose, mouth and skin, and are thought of as much more than just these body organs. For example, your sense of hearing moves out through your ears until it comes into contact with a sound vibration – it then bounces back and reports this impression to your mind. This is the reason many yogis practice pratyahara when sitting to meditate: attempting to withdraw the senses from the outside world by focusing on an internal point, such as the breath or a silently repeated mantra.

Whether you meditate or not, when all your senses are in harmony, properly nourished and regularly cleansed, you will feel healthier and more at peace. Unfortunately, the senses often behave like wild horses. Unless under the intelligent control of a firm driver – a strong mind – they attempt to pull you in various directions simultaneously. You may know you shouldn't eat a chocolate, but the cravings of your tongue often win out over the attempted logic and guidance of a perhaps not very disciplined mind. This lack of control can be particularly apparent when the mind and senses are cloudy, and in need of purification. With regular practice of the cleansing exercises in this book you should notice after a while that your self-control starts to strengthen and your mind becomes less distracted by sense impressions. Your physical, mental and emotional palate will clear and you will find that you crave an increasingly pure inner and outer environment.

"When you have cleansed your body, purified your mind and are able to control your senses, the joyful awareness that you need to realise your inner Self also comes." Patanjali's *Yoga Sutra*, 2–41

SITTING FOR MEDITATION

Cleansing techniques provide not only a firm foundation for the health of your physical body, they are also your doorway to deeper states of yoga and meditation. Meditation is considered the "king" or "crowning jewel" of yoga practice. When you meditate, prana is said to flow freely through the central energy channel of the nadi system, the sushumna (see page 18).

But to be able to meditate effectively you must first be able to sit comfortably in a balanced position for a length of time. The tranquility of your mind is dependent on the stability of your body, and when sitting for meditation, it is important to be able to assume a pose that encourages a feeling of spaciousness and clarity. If you feel compressed or constricted rather than aligned yet relaxed, it is difficult to experience your heart opening and consciousness expanding as you meditate.

When the cleansing exercises in this book ask you to sit in a meditation pose, choose one of the three positions that follow, sitting on a mat or folded blanket (a hard floor can soon hurt your feet and ankles). Then follow the guidelines for sitting (see opposite).

There are only three further suggestions I can offer for a successful yoga-cleansing meditation: practise, practise – and practise!

SIMPLE CROSS-LEGGED TAILOR POSE: SUKHASANA

This is the best sitting position to facilitate inward focus and stop energy from "leaking" – your legs form an infinity symbol, which conserves prana energy.

1 Sit with your legs crossed in front of you. If your knees are higher than your pelvis try raising your buttocks by sitting on a cushion or rolled-up blanket (but not too high, or your back will over-arch).

2 Check whether your knees are touching the ground. If not, support them with cushions or rolled-up blankets.

KNEELING ON YOUR HEELS: VAJRASANA

The pose commonly used in Zen meditation. If you find it difficult to sit directly on your heels, place a cushion, rolled-up blanket or yoga block between your buttocks and heels, or use a kneeling bench.

1 Kneel with your knees and feet together (or slightly apart), buttocks on your heels.

2 Make sure the front of your shins and feet contact the ground and your buttocks rest on your heels, cushion or bench.

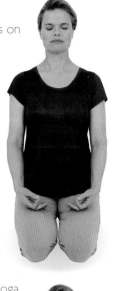

SITTING ON A CHAIR

Choose this option if you dislike sitting on the floor or can't bend your knees for an extended length of time. Choose a straight-backed chair with a firm seat.

1 Sit with your hips and buttocks on the seat of the chair and your thighs off the seat. Do not lean against the back of the chair; keep your body parallel to it. Place your feet flat on the floor (don't cross your ankles).

2 If your knees are higher than your pelvis, place a folded blanket or yoga block under your buttocks. If your feet don't reach the floor, rest them firmly on a cushion or block.

GUIDELINES FOR SITTING

- Sit up straight, but relaxed. If you slump forward (or lie down) you may fall asleep. If you sit up too rigidly, you create tension in the body.
- Let your spine be erect and perpendicular to the ground but maintain its natural curves. Then energy can travel up your spine and your breath be full. A bent spine impedes the movement of your diaphragm and ribcage, making it difficult to breathe deeply.
- Keep your chin parallel to the ground; imagine a fine thread lifting the top of your head and a thread attached to the centre of your breastbone keeping your chest upright.
- Align your body left and right; don't lean to one side or the other.
- Roll your shoulders forward and back 3–4 times. Then, keeping the shoulders relaxed, draw your shoulderblades slightly together and slide them down toward your waist. This counteracts round-shouldered habits acquired from sitting at a computer that hinder deep breathing.

HOW TO USE THIS BOOK

The best way to read this book is to dip in regularly and try out whichever practices appeal to you, rather than feeling that you need to read it from cover to cover. The six chapters at the heart of the book (Chapters 1–6) focus on ways to cleanse the five senses and the mind, offering ways to purify them literally and also mentally and spiritually, by working on the chakra linked to the sense.

The chapter on **Clarifying Your Vision** (see pages 28–49) offers techniques to cleanse and strengthen your physical eyes as well as your ajna (brow) chakra, often referred to as the "third eye", alongside several yoga balancing poses that hone your visual focus.

Enhancing Your Communication (see pages 50–69) suggests ways to enhance your sense of hearing and unblock your vishuddha (throat) chakra, which governs the energy of communication. The cleansing practices in this chapter include working with sound (Mantra, see page 62–3) and choosing to spend some time in voluntary silence (Mouna, see page 61).

Breathing More Deeply (see pages 70–89) presents techniques to cleanse your respiratory system as well as your muladhara (root) chakra, which controls your sense of smell. This chapter contains some of the best-known yoga cleansing exercises, such as Neti (see page 74), clearing out the nasal passages with a saline solution, and Kapalabhati (see page 76) which purifies using the rapid movement of air in and out of the lungs.

Nourishing Yourself (see pages 90–111) recommends a healthy purifying diet based around plant foods that calm the mind and reduce the negative effects of a stressful lifestyle. Along with ways to enhance your sense of taste are techniques to cleanse your entire digestive system. There are also suggestions for fasts to practise regularly and with the changing seasons.

Strengthening Your Connection with Others (see pages 112–131) introduces techniques to heighten your sense of touch and enhance the health of your skin. It also looks at the energetic centre of your body, where life tends to "touch" or inspire you, at the anahata (heart) chakra.

The chapter entitled **Simplifying Your Life** (see pages 132–149) provides ways to purify and fill your mind with positive thoughts, alongside techniques to clear your ajna (brow) chakra and your living and working environments.

In the final section of the book, entitled **Cleansing Routines** (see pages 150–55), you will find daily, weekly and seasonal sequences to help you fit the cleansing practices in the book into your life, plus ways to adapt them to suit your individual needs and preferences.

INTEGRATING CLEANSING INTO YOUR LIFE

It's easiest to cleanse body, mind and spirit when life doesn't feel overly complicated or cluttered. To keep things as simple as possible, before beginning to practise cleansing exercises make two lists: one of things that are important to you, and the second of tasks you could put on the back burner. Use these lists to set some long-term goals for ways to simplify your life. This enhances your ability to cleanse different aspects of life, from your environment and actions to your emotions, thoughts and attitudes.

Then act on these goals. Begin each week by writing a cleansing "intention" (*sankalpa*) describing the purifying techniques you will do. Make the statement active and positive, commit to an exact technique and amount of practice and avoid vague expressions. This helps to fix a firm image in your mind of you doing the practice.

Sample sankalpa: "This week I will do Neti each morning after brushing my teeth. Then I will do 3 rounds of Kapalabhati, 10 rounds of Alternate Nostril Breathing before sitting for 20 minutes for Heart-cleansing Meditation. Then I will write my journal for 10 minutes".

CLEANSING THROUGHOUT THE DAY

Feel free to supplement the routines throughout this book with the simple but invaluable activities listed below to further purify and clarify your life.

- Clear your desk, kitchen and work space before leaving it.
- Purify your air by ventilating rooms, changing air filters and using natural furnishings.
- Raise indoor plants to cleanse the air and amplify the concentration of prana.
- Select wisely from all the food, emotion and thought options available to you.
- Eat more organic and locally grown foods.
- Remove one potentially negative item from your diet weekly, noticing the effects.
- Decrease alcohol consumption if you drink, and if you smoke take steps to quit.
- Try not to gossip or spread negative opinions and judgements.
- Resolve to say what you mean in as non-hurtful a way as possible.
- Try to be aware of emotions and ideas you tend to "sweep under the carpet".
- Enjoy a period of introspection in the evening and ask yourself how transparent your communications were during the day.
- When home alone do not turn on the TV or music; enjoy the purity of silence for at least an hour each day.
- Notice how your thoughts and emotions are disturbed by violent conflict in the media.
- Take a regular yoga class and practise at home to increase the benefits of all the cleansing techniques in the book.

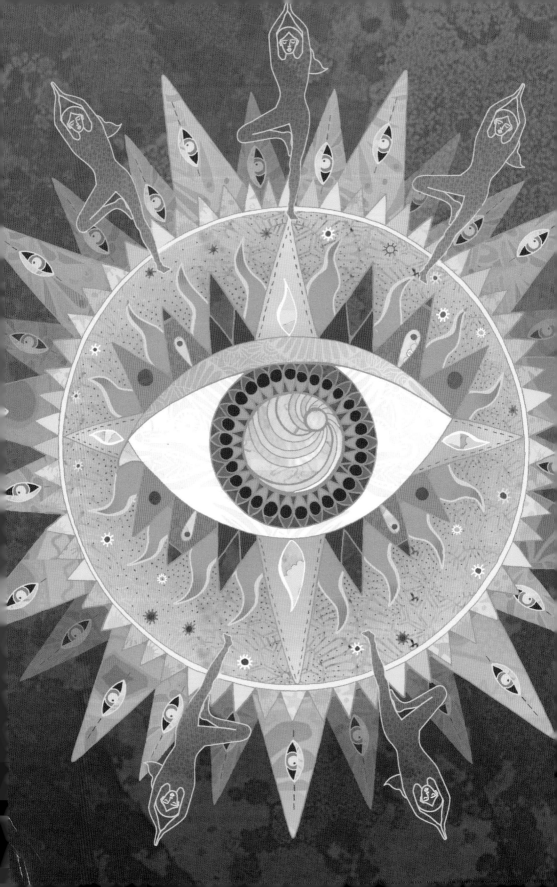

1
CLARIFYING YOUR VISION

FOR INCREASED CONCENTRATION AND INSIGHT

"You are not able to behold me with your own eyes;
I give you the divine eye, behold my lordly yoga."
Bhagavad Gita, 11.8

"...the common eye sees only the outside of things, and judges by that,
but the seeing eye pierces through and reads the heart and the soul..."
Mark Twain, *Personal Recollections of Joan of Arc*

PURIFYING YOUR SIGHT
– AND WAYS OF SEEING

Yoga teaches new ways of seeing and relating to the world. This chapter deals with ways of cleansing your sense of sight. You begin on a physical level with exercises to relax tension and build flexibility and range of motion, then move on to clarify the inner eye with practices that cultivate peace and a wider vision of what is really important in life.

THE SENSE OF SIGHT IN YOGA

Many of us take our sense of sight for granted. For example, you might try practising yoga with eyes closed, but even the simplest poses usually require some orientation by sight. It's often said that vision rules the brain: there are more neurons dedicated to sight than the other four senses put together. When your eyes are open, vision accounts for two-thirds of the electrical activity of the brain, which is why closing your eyes encourages relaxation and helps you fall asleep and also why the fastest way to make yourself concentrate on something is to look at it. Eye focus, *drishti*, is important in yoga practice.

EFFECTS OF CLEANSING YOUR SIGHT

While insight and inner peace may be the ultimate purpose of all yoga practices, many yoga cleansing techniques also bring about an improvement in eyesight. Perhaps surprisingly, it's not exercises that strengthen the eye muscles that seem to have greatest effect on vision; cleansing and relaxation appear to contribute more strongly to eye health, as well as movements that bring circulation to the face, neck and shoulders (see pages 32–35). As you age your eyes tend to get locked into habitual patterns and lose flexibility, making it increasingly difficult to focus on objects at varying distances. To preserve visual agility, this chapter includes cleansing Drishti (see page 46) as well as the ancient practice of staring at a candle flame, (Tratak, see pages 36–37). Mentioned in the 15th-century *Hatha Yoga Pradipika*, Tratak cleanses the tear ducts and sinuses while promoting concentration. Other yoga treatises recommend inner gazing, fixing the closed eyes on a point between the eyebrows as in Shambhavi Mudra (see page 47) to cleanse and cultivate deep peace. In addition to close and inner gazing, yoga texts mention the eye cleansing and strengthening brought about by a middle gaze achieved through balancing exercises, such as Tree Pose, Banyan Tree Pose, Dancing Siva Pose and Eagle Pose (see pages 40–43).

The eyes need darkness to recover from the stress of light and movement; the simplest way to de-stress them is to relax while covering your eyes (see Palming, page 33). Recipes for refreshing eyewashes are also included in this chapter (see pages 38–39).

SIGHT AND YOUR ENERGY BODY

Yoga focusing exercises help to purify and remove blockages from the nadi channels through which the energy yogis refer to as prana flows (see page 18). This chapter includes an exercise to cleanse the chitra nadi channel running between the ajna (brow) and heart (anahata) chakras (see page 45), making it more radiant, as well as a meditation to introduce the seven main chakra centres located along the sushumna channel (see page 48). There is a technique to enhance your brow chakra (see page 36) plus a light visualization that allows you to run a cleanse on all your chakras in turn or one in particular (see page 49).

SEEING MORE WIDELY

The eyes are often referred to as windows of the soul. You unthinkingly open them wide and soften them to show you are happy – and open them even wider but tensed when angry. You probably squint when you feel upset and appear unable to open them fully when sad. By looking at your eyes others gain an insight into your inner world – just as you look to their eyes for similar guidance. As the exercises in this chapter help cleanse, strengthen and relax your visual apparatus and keep your eyes looking clear, you will find that increasingly you inspire trust and communication is enhanced.

Ultimately, you see what your mind thinks you should see. Another consequence of practising the cleansing techniques in this chapter is that you free your mind of limitations and allow yourself to notice the bigger picture. With mental clarity and a cleansed perception come new possibilities – you may discover a talent for healing, for example – and the chance to choose how you experience the world and how the world sees you.

BENEFITS OF CLEANSING YOUR SENSE OF SIGHT

• Improves your eyesight and enhances peripheral vision.
• Develops concentration and calms the mind.
• Relieves eyestrain caused by prolonged computer use.
• Upgrades your ability to visualize and increases spiritual insight.

EYE EXERCISES
To strengthen your vision

Exercising the eyes helps to clear away the negative effects of daily stress, strain and environmental toxins, such as intense artificial light. These techniques are especially beneficial if you spend long periods of time reading or working at a computer. The cleansing effects not only improve your physical vision, but help you to become more focused and can bring spiritual insight, greatly enhancing a yoga practice. Practise these exercises sitting on a chair (preferably with a straight back), kneeling or sitting cross-legged on the ground, keeping your spine straight and head lifted (see pages 24–25)

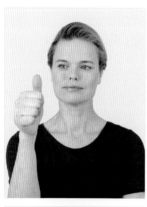

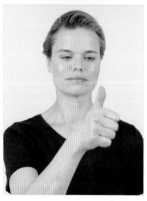

STRENGTHEN AND CLEANSE THE EYES

This first series of exercises increases circulation to the eyes and warms up the muscles around them.

1 Up and down: Open your eyes wide; imagine 'popping' them out of your head. Keeping your head and neck still, look up as high as you can, then down. Repeat 10–15 times. Then close your eyes to relax them for a moment.

2 Right and left: Raise your left arm, thumb pointing up and elbow straight. Open your eyes wide and focus on your thumbnail. Slowly move your hand to the left, following the nail with your eyes (see pictures, right). The slower you move, the harder your eyes have to work and the greater the benefits. Move the hand out as far as you can see without moving your head. Just as slowly, return your hand and eyes to centre. Change arms and repeat to the right. Repeat 2–3 times on each side. Close and relax your eyes.

3 Diagonal: Making gentle fists and, straightening your elbows, raise your right arm, thumb pointing up, and lower your left, thumb pointing out slightly. Open your eyes as wide as possible. Without moving your head, look up at your right thumb, down at your left, and up to the right again. Repeat 8–10 times. Change arms and repeat. Rest your eyes for a few moments.

PRACTICE TIPS

- Remove glasses or contact lenses before starting eye exercises.
- Perform all the movements slowly and gently.
- Try to move just your eyes, not your head.
- If your eyes start to water while practising, count it as an especially successful cleanse.

RELAX THE EYES

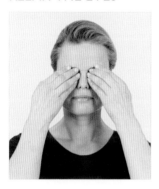

Practise this recovery relaxation sequence between other exercises and at the end of your session.

1 Blinking: Open your eyes and blink quickly 10–20 times. Then close your eyes and relax for 3–5 breaths.

2 Palming: Close your eyes and rub your hands together vigorously until they feel warm. Then cup your hands over your eyes so that they cover them (see picture, right). Keep your neck long. Once your eyes have relaxed, drop your hands and blink a few times.

IMPROVE EYE FLEXIBILITY

This series of exercises encourages the eye muscles to work in non-habitual ways. Practising regularly helps to preserve a full range of movement.

1 Circles: Open your eyes wide and look up. Very slowly, rotate your eyes in a clockwise direction; make sure you cover the whole circumference of the widest circle possible with your eyes. After 3–5 rotations, repeat the rotation anti-clockwise.

2 Infinity symbols: Extend your left arm, thumb pointing upward. Following your thumbnail with your eyes, slowly move your arm up (as high as you can see your thumb) then circle it to the left, down and back to the centre. Change arms and repeat to the right. Change arms again until you have "drawn" 3–5 infinity symbols in the air. Repeat in the opposite direction, circling to the right first.

3 Spirals: Bring one hand to your waist, thumb pointing upward. Follow your thumbnail with your eyes as you circle your hand away from your body making a horizontal movement that becomes an upward-moving spiral. When you can no longer see the thumb, spiral downward, changing hands if your hand gets tired.

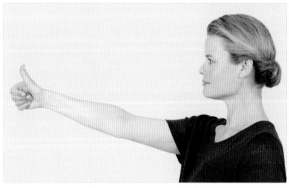
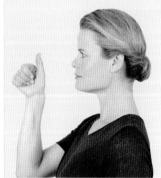

CHANGE FOCUS MORE EASILY

This counters the first eye problem many people have and is useful if you wear glasses.

1 Focus on tip of nose: Open your eyes wide. Extend one arm; raise your hand in front of your nose, thumb up. Focusing on your thumbnail, bend your elbow and move your thumb slowly toward the tip of your nose, as close as you can maintain focus, then away. Repeat 5–10 times.

2 Focus on third eye: Lift your arm 6–8cm (3-4 inches). Focusing on the nail, slowly bring your thumb toward the point between your eyebrows, then out again. Repeat 5–10 times.

3 Long-distance to close-up: Sit outdoors or by a window. Pick a point in the distance, preferably on the horizon; this is your long-distance focus point. Extend your arm, thumb up. Look at your thumbnail, then the long-distance point. Alternate your focus rhythmically between the two 10–15 times. Relax by palming (see page 33), breathing deeply.

4 Three focus points: Extend one arm, thumb up, and bring your other thumb 15cm (6in) in front of your nose – the thumbnails are your middle and close-up focal points. Alternate between them 10–15 times. Then shift focus between the close-up and long-distance points 10–15 times. Finish by relaxing your eyes (see page 33).

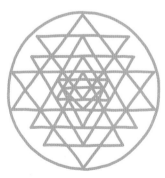

STRENGTHEN EACH EYE

Before starting this exercise, place a geometric pattern, such as a yantra (left) at arm's distance from your face.

1 Cover one eye with your hand. Trace the shape of each of the patterns with your uncovered eye. If you are using the popular Sri Yantra, first trace the 5 upward-pointing triangles, then the 4 downward-pointing ones.

2 Change eyes and repeat the exercise.

BUILD RANGE OF MOTION

This somatic-yoga practice helps you focus on the inner experience of the exercise while exploring the brain-muscle-neurological connection. It may take a few repetitions to get used to, but strengthens the eye muscles and increases their range of motion. If you find the leg position uncomfortable, sit on a chair, feet flat on the floor, hands resting on your thighs.

1 Sit on the ground with your left knee forward and bent, left foot touching your right thigh. Bend your right knee back, heel near your right buttock. Place your left palm on the floor near your left hip with your fingers spread wide, making a firm base. Rest your right hand on your right thigh.

1a Keeping your chest and shoulders still, turn your head to look over your left shoulder. Then your right shoulder. Repeat 3–5 times, then return it to centre.

2 Maintaining the leg position, place your left hand on your right shoulder, elbow resting on your chest (see picture, top). Slowly rotate your torso and head left and look over your left shoulder. Without moving your torso or shoulders, turn your head to look over your right shoulder. Turn the head slowly left and right 3–5 times in a full range of motion. Finish with head and shoulders to the left; hold a moment.

3 Keeping shoulders and upper body to the left, turn your head to the right. Then rotate your torso to the right as you turn your head left. Repeat this criss-cross 3–5 times on each side, ending with shoulders to the left and head to the right.

4 Continue looking right with your eyes as you turn your head left (see picture, middle). Then turn your head right as you turn your eyes to look left. Repeat the head and eyes criss-cross 3–5 times, then bring your head and eyes back to a central position.

5 Now bring your hands onto your knees. Lift your head as you arch your shoulders and back; look up. Then round your back and neck so you curl inward and look down. Repeat 3–5 times.

5a Repeat the up and down movement, but bring your eyes into opposition. As you arch up and back look down (see picture, bottom). Then look up as your head, chest and shoulders curl down. Repeat 3–5 times then return to a neutral position.

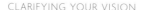

STEADY GAZING: TRATAK
To increase your focus

A powerful yet deceptively simple exercise, Tratak is one the six classical yoga cleansing exercises or kriyas (see page 15). It purifies the eyes, tear ducts and sinuses while helping to strengthen your eyesight and bring a fresh supply of blood to the forehead. Energetically, it works as a powerful psychic cleanser for the brow (ajna) chakra (see page 19), decreasing lethargy and increasing your powers of discernment. It makes an effective part of a meditation toolkit because it promotes intense concentration.

Tratak stimulates the pineal gland. Located at the centre of the brain, between the two hemispheres, this smallest member of the endocrine system produces melatonin, the hormone that regulates sleep patterns, our internal body clock and seasonal cycles. So by promoting more effective sleep hygiene, this technique is a great aid for sleep-related disorders and issues with the circadian biological clock. Regular practice can be especially effective in the winter months, when reduced levels of sunlight contribute to Seasonal Affective Disorder (SAD). Avoid practising Tratak if you have epilepsy, and practise with care if you have an eye problem such as glaucoma.

FOCUS ON A CANDLE FLAME

Known as *Diya Tratak*, this method uses the flame of a candle as a focal point. It works best in a darkened room. Remove glasses or contact lenses before starting the exercise, and if you feel any strain or tension in your eye muscles stop practising.

1 Place a lit candle an arm's distance in front of you so that your eyes and the flame are on approximately the same horizontal plane, but with the candle slightly lower. Choose a place without draughts to keep the flame steady and unflickering.

2 Sit in a comfortable meditation position with your spine straight and head erect (see pages 24–25). Allow your hands to rest comfortably in your lap or on your thighs.

3 Open your eyes wide and look deeply into the flame, trying not to blink or move your eyeballs. Release any tension in your face and eye muscles. Hold the gaze for approximately 1 minute, noticing how the flame has several rings of differing colours. If your eyes cross or you see multiple images, refocus and return to a relaxed gaze (see picture, right).

4 Close your eyes to allow the muscles to relax. Then repeat the alternate gaze and relaxation several times.

5 Finally, close your eyes and visualize the flame at the point between your eyebrows.

Try not to concentrate on the physical glow that arises when you stimulate the optic nerve with a bright light. Instead use your mind's eye to draw a mental picture of the flame, including all its rings and colours.

6 When you have finished, splash your eyes with cold water. As you become more practised, gradually increase the amount of time you hold the gaze to 5, 10 or even 20 minutes. Stop when tears stream down your face.

> "Gaze with motionless eyes at a minute object with your mind concentrated until tears come. This is called *trataka* by the gurus. By *trataka*, sloth and all diseases of the eyes are removed. So it should be carefully preserved, as you would a golden box." *Hatha Yoga Pradipika*, 2.31–32

FOCUS ON AN IMAGE

You can also practise Tratak by concentrating your gaze on any static visual or shape that stands out strongly against its background. The following are popular – choose any that appeal to you:

- Black spot on a white background, known as *Bindu Tratak*.
- A *yantra* (see page 34), a mystical symbol in the form of a geometric diagram, for example the geometric forms associated with the five elements of yoga philosophy (earth, water, fire, air and space) or the various chakras (see page 19).
- Staring into your eyes in a mirror (*Darpan Tratak*).

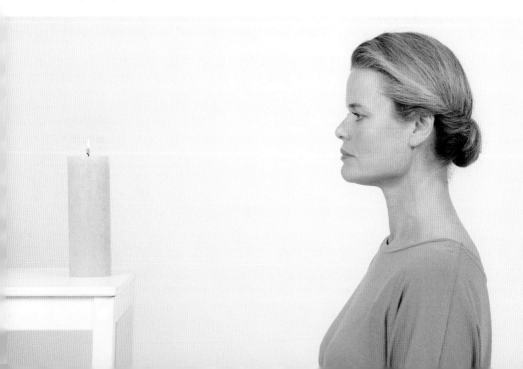

BATHING THE EYES
To refresh your outlook

Cleaning the eyes is a useful antidote to the drying effects of central heating and air conditioning, and spending hours at a screen, which can cause the tear ducts to become congested. Some opthalmologists recommend a few drops of well diluted "tearless" baby shampoo to clear debris from the tear ducts and combat dry eyes and eyelid disorders like inflammation. Many yogis prefer herbal eyewashes said to enhance the eyes' ability to lubricate themselves. Eye washes are not recommended for injuries to the eyes or eye area. For conjunctivitis, glaucoma or cataracts, consult your doctor or healthcare professional.

REJUVENATING EYE COMPRESS
This simplified variation of the Ayurvedic treatment *Netra Tarpana* is used to rejuvenate the eyes and counteract dryness. You will need a little castor oil, heated ghee or honey, a face cloth and an old towel.

1 Remove make-up; place the towel on your pillow.

2 Dip the cloth in the oil, ghee or honey; fold into a compress. Lie with your head on the pillow and apply the eye compress to your closed eyes for 20 minutes.

MORNING HERBAL EYEWASH
This recipe makes a slightly astringent eye-wash that doubles as an excellent skin toner.

1 tsp eyebright herb; if unable to source or concerned about contraindications,
   substitute water
100ml/3½fl oz/scant ½ cup boiling water
50ml/2 fl oz/scant ¼ cup rosewater
130ml/4 fl oz/½ cup witch-hazel extract (alcohol-free)

1 Place the eyebright in a cup, cover with boiling water and allow to steep for 10 minutes. Strain, discard the herbs and allow the liquid to cool.

2 Combine this eyebright tisane with the rosewater and witch hazel; refrigerate in a sterilized dark glass bottle.

3 Apply on a cotton pad as part of your morning routine.

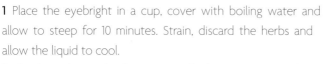

CLEANSING THE THIRD EYE

While focusing on the brow (ajna) and crown (sahasrara) chakras (see page 19), this simple treatment stimulates a cleansing response in your entire energetic system.

1 Fill a sink or large bowl with cold water. Tie back long hair, if you have it. Place your forehead and the front part of your head in the water.

2 Hold for about 1 minute (choose whether to keep your eyes closed or blink in the water). Be sure to dry your hair properly afterwards.

TRIPHALA EYE BATH

This quick and stimulating flush is an excellent way to ease tired, irritated and dry or red eyes. Some yogis report that washing the eyes with triphala water seems to make the world look more beautiful energetically: colours appear brighter, the sky looks clearer. You will need triphala powder, an eye bath and some muslin cloth or a paper coffee filter.

1 Place ½ tsp triphala powder in a cup and fill with boiling water. Stir, leave for a few hours, then strain through the muslin or coffee filter paper into a glass or cup.

2 Fill the eye bath ¾ full with the liquid. Lean your head forward and fix the rim of the bath around one eye. It is designed to fit around the eye and create a gentle suction so the liquid doesn't run down your face.

3 Holding the eye bath in place, turn your head up so your eye is immersed in the triphala water. Slowly blink a few times. Don't worry if it stings a little. Your eye will soon relax enough to open, but if you find it too uncomfortable, stop and rinse with tepid water.

4 Bathe your eye for 2–5 minutes. When comfortable, try simple eye exercises, moving your eyeball slowly right and left, up and down, diagonally, clockwise and anti-clockwise.

5 Remove the bath, dry your eye and repeat with the other eye. Then relax for a few minutes. Avoid screens for at least 30 minutes following the treatment.

THE CLEANSING POWER OF TRIPHALA

Triphala is a formulation of three Indian herbs valued in Ayurveda as an antioxidant and for nourishing and rejuvenating tissue. Some yogis drink remaining triphala water from an eye bath, but avoid if you are pregnant, breastfeeding or taking blood-thinning medication.

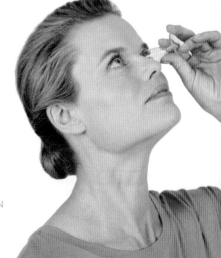

TREE POSE: VRIKSHASANA
To steady your vision

To clarify your powers of visual concentration, try this classic yoga pose, which also strengthens physical and mental balance. Begin by trying to develop a steady foundation and connection with the earth, then gradually allow yourself to "grow" upward.

1 Stand tall with your knees straight and arms relaxed at your sides. Feel your bodyweight spread evenly over both your feet. This is Mountain Pose (Tadasana). Close your eyes and become aware of the exchange of energy between your body and the earth. Then try to sense the energy spreading up through your knees and thighs and into your trunk.

2 Once you feel balanced and grounded, bend your right knee and place your right foot flat against the inside of your left thigh, as high up as possible.

3 Keeping your left leg straight and steady, bring your palms together at your chest. Fix your gaze on a point on the wall or ceiling approximately 1m (3ft) ahead of you.

4 Slowly straighten your arms and raise them overhead, palms together (see picture, below right). As you hold the pose, visualize your left foot sending roots into the ground. Allow the gravity of the earth to help you stand firm, but feel your arms lifting you up. Hold for 10 seconds, then lower your foot and arms.

5 Repeat on the other leg. Increase the hold gradually to 1 minute on each side.

SIMPLE VARIATION

If you cannot bring your foot high on the opposite thigh, place it wherever it is comfortable on the inner leg. Keep your palms together in front of your breastbone in prayer position, Namaste Mudra.

PRACTICE TIP

- Start with your side 15cm (6in) from a wall. Place your hand on the wall and come into the pose. When ready, bring your hands together overhead.

BANYAN TREE POSE: VATYASANA
For uplifting rooting

Balancing exercises like this challenging pose heighten the cleansing power of intense concentration because you can only hold them for as long as you can maintain your focus. When first practising this pose, try standing with your right side beside a wall, but not touching it, for balance.

Always practise under the guidance of an experienced teacher.

1 Stand tall with your knees straight and arms relaxed at your sides in Mountain Pose (Tadasana, see opposite). Bend your right knee and place your right foot on top of your left thigh, as close to the hip as possible.

2 Fix your gaze on a still point opposite you, then slowly bend your left knee and slowly and carefully lower your body towards the ground. Keep your back upright and slide your eyes down the wall until your right knee reaches the floor, or as close to the floor as you feel comfortable to go. If your knee can reach the floor, you should be supported on your right knee and left foot. If you are not able to put your knee on the ground, simply lower it as close to the ground as you can.

3 Bring your palms together in front of your breastbone in prayer position, Namaste Mudra. Hold whichever version of the pose you are able to achieve for approximately 10 seconds, keeping your gaze steady.

4 Release the leg position, then slowly stand up and turn (so that your left side is near the wall, if you are using a wall) and repeat the pose with your left foot on your right thigh. Gradually increase the hold to 30 seconds on each side with practice.

VARIATION

Though simpler than a full Banyan Tree Pose, this variation is still challenging and should only be attempted under guidance from an experience teacher.

Start the position from kneeling, then bring your right foot around and place on top of your left thigh while keeping both knees on the ground for support. Bring your hands into Namaste Mudra (see picture, right) and hold the pose for 10 seconds, then return to a kneeling position and repeat with the opposite leg.

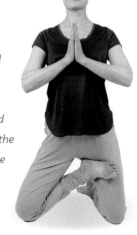

DANCING SIVA POSE: NATARAJASANA
To develop inner poise

Mental clarity, cleansed perception and a sense of lightness arise naturally as you develop inner poise. Balancing poses help the process by encouraging greater coordination between your muscles and brain. This beautiful asana, named after the cosmic dancer, the Hindu god Siva, is sometimes referred to as *devadutāsana*, the "flying angel", and with regular practice, your body will become as light and graceful as your purified mind as your hip flexors open and strengthen. If you find it difficult to balance, practise within touching distance of a wall.

1 Stand tall with your feet parallel to each other; fix your gaze firmly on a point approximately 2m (6ft) in front of you. Bend your right knee, taking your right foot back and up toward your right buttock. Reach back with your right hand and take hold of your right ankle.

2 Stretch your left arm straight up, alongside your left ear. Imagine your body is one solid piece from your bent right knee up to the fingers on your left hand.

3 Gradually begin to lift your bent knee and try to bring the right foot as high and as far from the right buttock as possible. As you do this, your entire body will tilt forward slightly.

4 Keep lifting your bent knee until your body is almost parallel with the ground. Balance in this position, breathing gently. Keep your arm straight and alongside your ear. Try to hold the position for 5 breaths. Let your inhalations and exhalations be slow and even.

5 Lift back to centre and lower your arm and leg. Repeat on the other side, gradually increasing the hold to 20 breaths on each side with practice.

EAGLE POSE: GARUDASANA
To open yourself to new possibilities

By twisting the arms and legs in this pose, you challenge the way your brain experiences your body, which cleanses your perception and feels refreshing. In Indian mythology, Garuda, for whom the pose is named, is the eagle-like bird that transports the Hindu god Vishnu. He is visualized as the golden-bodied lord of the sky who symbolizes freedom and being open to new possibilities. Practising his pose brings about a joyous sense of liberation and harmony while improving balance and coordination.

    If you have a knee injury practise eagle pose carefully and ease out of the pose if you feel any pain.

1 Stand firmly with feet parallel to each other; bend both knees slightly and fix your gaze on a point 2m (6ft) in front of you.

2 Shift your weight to your left foot. Lift your right leg and cross it over your left at the thigh, hooking your right toes behind your left calf.

3 Keeping your back straight, bend your right elbow and bring your arm in front of your chest, fingers pointing up. Bend your left elbow and bring it under your right elbow. Keep your elbows stacked on top of each other and try to bring your palms together, like an eagle's beak. Hold for 5–10 slow breaths. To deepen the pose, bend your knees and slide your body down in a straight line so you sit closer to the ground; try not to lean forward.

4 Release the pose, shake out your shoulders and legs. Repeat on the other side.

VARIATION: WITH FOOT DOWN
Cross your right thigh over your left, placing the tips of your right toes on the floor outside your left foot. Continue as for the main pose.

GAZING INTO THE VOID: BHUCHARI MUDRA
To promote concentration

This powerfully cleansing hand gesture helps to free your mind of perceived limitations by promoting intense concentration. Used as a meditation technique, it promotes feelings of peace and of being at one with the universe. With practice, you become better able to see the "big picture". If you wear glasses or contact lenses, it is best to remove them before practising this exercise.

Physically, Bhuchari Mudra is valued for cleansing the tear ducts, sinuses and frontal region of the head while strengthening the nerve centres in the neck and eyes. On a more subtle level, it purifies and stimulates the throat (vishuddha) chakra (see page 19) as well as a minor energy centre known as *soma* chakra located just above the back of the soft palate. This chakra is valued by yogis for promoting graceful ageing by assisting the processes by which the body retains its vitality and stamina. Practise daily.

1 Sit with your back straight and place the thumbnail of one hand flat against the ridge between your nose and upper lip. Gently curl your index, middle and ring fingers into your palm; stretch your little finger out straight.

2 Open your eyes wide and stare at the tip of your little finger, trying to blink as infrequently as possible. Try to relax any tension in your face. After a few moments, your eyes may start to tear. Do not stop; this cleanses your eyes, tear ducts and sinuses. Continue starring at your little finger for 3–5 minutes.

3 Now, without moving your gaze, drop your hand. Do not allow your eyes to follow your hand; continue to look intently at the point where the tip of your little finger was. Aim to gaze into the void in this way for 15–20 minutes, keeping your head erect and eyes steady; don't allow them to cross.

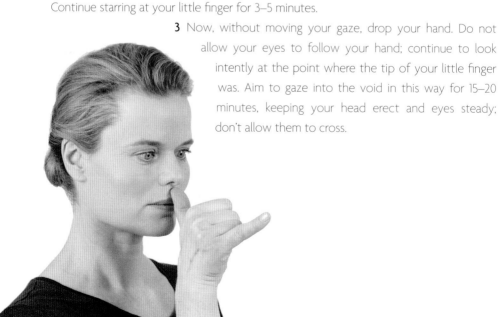

CHITRA MERIDIAN VISUALIZATION
To raise your energy

The major meridians of the subtle body – the ida, pingala and sushumna channels or nadis through which the subtle energy yogis call prana travels – are often mentioned in yoga (see page 18). But several ancient texts claim that the central sushumna nadi has various degrees of subtleness and that there is a pathway here known as *chitra* that is even more refined and pure in nature. The Sanskrit word *chitra* means "bright", "clear", "radiant" or "luminous". This visualization cleanses this channel of the subtle energy body.

If this energy pathway is sufficiently purified that prana channels through it, you will have a bright and quiet experience of raised energy. This is considered by yogis to be a first step in developing extraordinary talents, such as the ability to heal or even telepathy. Some texts claim that chitra emanates from the heart, and from there extends both up to the crown chakra and down to the sacral chakra. This may be interpreted to mean that you always have a choice of direction in which to channel your energy.

1 You can practise sitting or lying down. Choose a comfortable position (for sitting positions, see pages 24–25) and close your eyes.

2 As you breathe in, visualize your breath as a light entering your body through the brow (ajna) chakra. Visualize the breath travelling down a silver tube that runs to your heart. See yourself breathing out through the heart.

3 Now visualize breathing in through your heart. The breath enters the silver tube and travels up to the brow chakra, where you breathe out.

4 Again breathe in through the brow chakra and out through the heart. Then breathe in through the heart and out through brow chakra. Continue in this way for 15–20 minutes. If you are lying down, you may find that you fall asleep and wake with your mind feeling especially cleansed and rejuvenated.

> "Chitra is the highest and most beloved by the yogis. Brilliant with five colours, it is in the centre of Sushumna. It is the most vital part of the body called the 'heavenly way'. It is the giver of Immortality. By contemplating on the chakras that exist in this nadi, the yogi destroys all sins and attains the highest bliss. It is the giver of moksha (liberation)." Swami Sivananda

FOCUSING THE EYES: DRISHTI
To purify inner vision

The practice of fixing your gaze on a point – Drishti – is a yoga cleansing discipline in itself, but also bolsters the purifying effects of other practices. When practising Drishti you stay in the present moment, stopping your attention from wandering by directing it to specific points, such as the tip of your nose or forehead. This removes blockages from the nadi energy channels (see page 18), stimulating the healing flow of the subtle energy yogis call prana. It also cleanses and equalizes energy in the chakras (see page 19).

Physically, the practice relieves tension and improves blood circulation to the frontal region of the head and brain. It helps you to hold yoga balancing poses (see pages 40–43) and draws the body into correct alignment. Practise Nasagra and Bhrumadhya Drishti first; they are preliminaries for Shambhavi Mudra (see opposite). It is best to practise Drishti under the guidance of an experienced teacher.

NASAL GAZE: NASAGRA DRISHTI

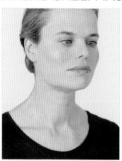

After you have perfected this technique, you will notice that your eyes stronger. Use in Lion's Yawn Pose (see page 56).

1 Sit in a comfortable meditation position, spine straight and head erect (see pages 24–25). Turn your gaze down and focus both eyes on the tip of your nose, eyelids half-closed. Hold for 10 seconds. Then close and relax your eyes.

2 Gradually build up the practice, stopping when your eyes feel strained, until you can hold the gaze for 1 minute.

FRONTAL GAZE: BHRUMADHYA DRISHTI

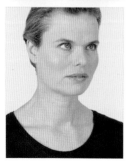

When you can practise nasal gaze without tension, try turning your eyes up toward the front of your brain, fixing your vision on the point between your eyebrows. Hold for 10 seconds only, then close and relax your eyes. Use this gaze in Fish Pose (Matsyasana) if you practise it, but prolonged practice is not recommended.

INNER GAZE: SHAMBHAVI MUDRA

In this purifying gaze you close the eyes and focus inward. If you can hold your attention here and become truly immersed, you will feel deep peace and experience your purest self, the aim of all forms of yoga practice.

1 Sit in a comfortable meditation position (see pages 24–25). Close your eyes; breathe gently through your nose. Bring your awareness to the parts of your body in contact with the ground: buttocks, legs and feet. Visualize roots growing into the earth. Inhaling, imagine drawing energy up from the earth. Exhaling, release impurities and negativity into the earth.

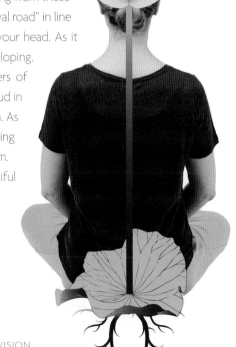

2 When ready, visualize a flower stem slowly growing from these roots up along the sushumna energy channel, or "royal road" in line with your spine. Picture the stalk growing toward your head. As it reaches the point behind your eyes, see a bud developing.

3 Direct your eyes inward as you use your powers of imagination and visualization. Gaze intently at the bud in the space behind the forehead. See it begin to open. As it slowly unfolds, the petals spread out and a sparkling white 1,000-petaled lotus flower gradually takes form.

4 Notice inside the flower a smaller, yet more beautiful shimmering multi-coloured 12-petalled lotus.

5 Continue gazing at the flower; notice a radiant ball of light forming within it. If it is faint, focus your attention and it will become more distinct.

6 Hold the image as long as is comfortable. Slowly open your eyes, blink and come to.

CHAKRA-AWARENESS MEDITATION
To connect to the cleansing power of chakras

We can use various visualization and meditation techniques to purify the chakras (see pages 18–19) in order to keep them open and fully operational. This ensures good physical, mental and emotional health, and determines how well you "inhabit" your physical body, the success of your relationships, and how much inner peace you are able to enjoy. But before you can start cleansing the chakras, you need to be able to experience these subtle energy centres. This exercise introduces you each chakra in turn, allowing you to experience it as a multi-dimensional ball of radiant energy and a conduit that conducts and transforms the subtle energy of prana into material form.

1 Sit in a comfortable meditation position, spine straight and head erect (see pages 24–25); do not lie down. Close your eyes; seal your lips, breathing gently through your nostrils.

2 After a few breaths, gradually make your breath longer, directing it downward. Continue lengthening your breath until you feel you are breathing into the base of your body.

3 As you inhale send your breath down along the front of your body. Exhaling, feel the breath moving up your spine from its base to the crown of your head. It may help to visualize your breath as a stream of bright white light. As you inhale the light moves down your front, and as you exhale, it moves up your back. Continue until the rhythm is regular.

4 As your breath moves up your back, try to experience the various energetic points that relate to the chakras. Slowly move your awareness in turn to:

- **Root (muladhara) chakra**: at the base of your body, the areas that come into contact with the ground when you sit down.
- **Sacral (swadhisthana) chakra**: in your sacral region, where the kidneys are located in the middle of your lower back.
- **Solar plexus (manipura) chakra**: at the solar plexus, the area above your naval and below your ribs.
- **Heart (anahata) chakra**: in the middle of your breastbone – sense your energetic heart, rather than your physical heart.
- **Throat (vishuddha) chakra**: at your throat.
- **Brow (ajna) chakra**: at the centre of your forehead, between your eyebrows.
- **Crown (sahasrara) chakra**: at the top of your head.

5 As you sit tuning into each of the energy centres, simply notice which ones you experience more strongly and which seem weaker.

CLEANSING YOUR CHAKRAS WITH LIGHT
To clarify your energy

One way of keeping the chakras (see pages 18–19) purified and open is to visualize light running through each one to clean, energize and balance it. This chakra-cleansing exercise takes just a few minutes. You may want to try it before a meditation session or yoga practice, or in the morning as part of your cleansing routine. You could run a daily general cleanse on all the chakras or, on some days, you may prefer to concentrate on cleansing one in particular. For example, if you feel you have an impurity in a certain chakra, spend more time running light through it.

1 Sit in a comfortable meditation position with your spine straight and head erect (see pages 24–25). Close your eyes and take a few slow deep breaths; feel the in-breath inflating your lower abdomen.

2 Gradually elongate the breath until you are breathing into the parts of your body that are in contact with the ground. Visualize yourself growing roots down deep into the earth. Remind yourself that roots have multiple jobs. They can ground you, and they can assist you in releasing waste products. With each exhalation, feel as though you are releasing what you no long need or want into the earth.

3 Once you feel fully grounded, bring your awareness to the top of your head; imagine a beautiful white or golden light rotating just above it. Visualize the light slowly entering your crown (sahasrara) chakra at the top of your head; notice whether or not you experience any physical sensations as this happens.

4 Move your awareness to your forehead. Visualize the light rotating clockwise to purify your brow (ajna) chakra.

5 Then move your awareness down to your throat; See the light picking up debris and carrying it away from your throat (vishuddha) chakra.

6 In the same way move your awareness down your body, to your heart (anahata) chakra, solar plexus (manipura) chakra, sacral (swadhisthana) chakra and root (muladhara) chakra. As you sit, working down through each chakra, simply visualize the same cleansing light whirling clockwise.

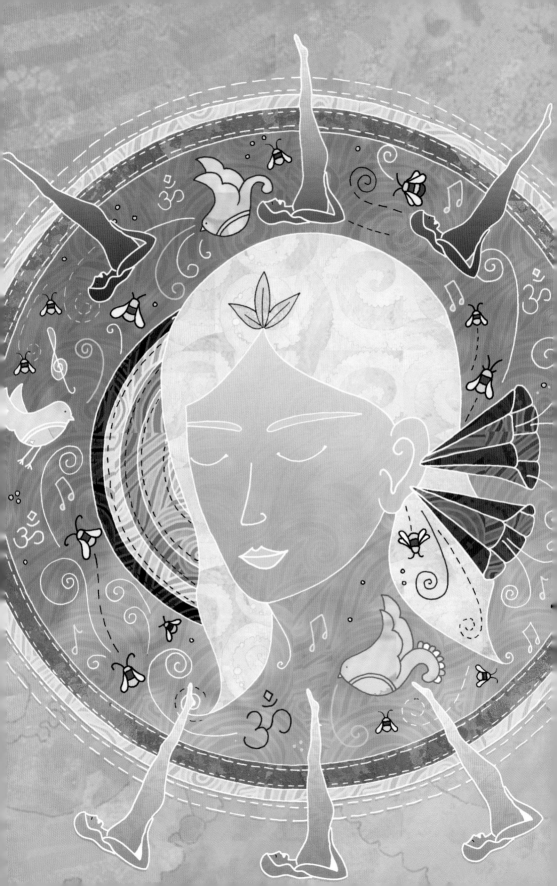

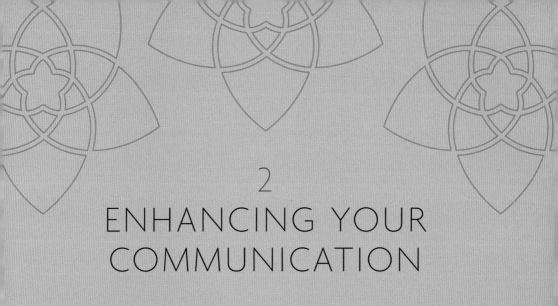

2
ENHANCING YOUR
COMMUNICATION

FOR GREATER SELF-EXPRESSION AND UNDERSTANDING

*"There is a difference between truly listening
and waiting for your turn to talk."*
Ralph Waldo Emerson

*"The most important thing in communication
is hearing what isn't being said."*
Anonymous

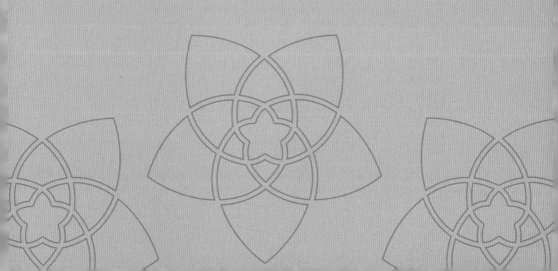

AUGMENTING YOUR HEARING – HOW YOU SOUND

Yoga often calls on the sense of hearing – while chanting or repeating mantras, when seeking silence in meditation or resting in moments of stillness through the day. In this chapter we cleanse this sense by tuning into different sound frequencies. This replenishes *ojas*, the basic physical energy of your body, or inner strength, while converting it into *tejas*, spiritual radiance. By doing so you find new ways to hear and trust your inner voice.

THE SENSE OF HEARING IN YOGA

Most people find it easier to concentrate using their hearing than any other sense. For example, it's difficult to bring to mind a particular taste or scent. But you can probably "hear" a song you loved as a teenager even if you haven't listened to it for years. In yoga classes, people often ask "Can I use a visual image to focus on?" You can, but it is more difficult than focusing on a sound. You might picture a red rose, for example, but find it soon turns pink in your mind's eye. It begins as a bud, starts to open, and then you see a garden of roses and remember someone sending roses for your birthday Sound doesn't usually shape-shift or morph in the same way; it is much more stable. In fact sound is such a fundamental yoga concept that it is said to have brought the world into being. The idea of *sabda-brahma* (creation by sound) may correlate to the Biblical phrase "In the beginning was the Word" and the Big Bang theory in science. This chapter takes such cosmological principles out of the realm of theory and puts them to work in a pragmatic way.

EFFECTS OF CLEANSING YOUR HEARING

In yoga theory, sound is regarded as a form of energy that manifests at four fundamental levels, with audible sound at the gross physical end of the spectrum and transcendental experience as the most subtle state. This chapter offers cleansing techniques for all levels:

1 Para: transcendental sound, or the primal substratum of thought and language. This undifferentiated potential sound corresponds to the initial vibration that brought the universe into being and unites everything. Purify your hearing on this highest level by meditating and practising: Chanting OM (see pages 62–63), Sagarbha (see page 82).

2 Pashyanti: telepathic sound or the universal level of thought that does not differentiate by naming. If we think about a flower, for example, each of us experiences it in non-verbal language. You can purify your vocal cords and mind on this subtle level by practising: Bhramari Pranayama with the help of Shanmukhi Mudra (see pages 54–55).

3 **Madhyama:** the mental vibration of thinking in language rather than images. We tend to select words through a mental prism clouded by preconceptions, sense impressions, emotions and past experiences. You can purify this level of hearing by practising: Ujjayi Pranayama (see pages 64–65) and by cleansing your chakras with sound (see page 67).

4 **Vaikhari:** the dense, audible sound of the spoken word, and most concrete state of sound. This is thought translated into the speech by which we communicate. Clean your ears to optimize hearing and purify your vocal cords by practising: oil baths (see page 66), Lion's Yawn Pose, Shoulderstand and neck exercises (see pages 56–59).

HEARING AND YOUR ENERGY BODY

Your throat (vishuddha) chakra (see page 19) governs your sense of hearing as well as your ability to speak and express yourself. When your throat and hearing apparatus are cleansed on all levels, you can express yourself more honestly and articulate your emotional needs openly, without fearing others' opinions. The exercises in this chapter remove blockages and tone the throat chakra, clearing barriers to communication, while Vishuddha Chakra Meditation (see pages 68–69) ensures the free-flow of artistic energy and a cleansing chakra sound bath (see page 67) tunes you into the wisdom of your inner voice.

THE POWER OF LISTENING

Communication is only partly about speaking and being heard. It also involves listening deeply to understand what someone is trying to tell you. Cultivating a period of silence each day (Mouna, see page 61) has a cleansing effect that helps you listen, while detoxing your language of negative expressions (see page 60) equips you to respond to others with compassion. Such purity of voice creates positive vibrations that transform relationships.

BENEFITS OF CLEANSING YOUR SENSE OF HEARING
• Improves your hearing and ability to focus in noisy environments.
• Develops concentration as you quiet your mind.
• Enhances your ability to communicate effectively.
• Strengthens the ability to tune into your inner rhythm and boosts spiritual motivation.

BEE BREATH: BHRAMARI PRANAYAMA
To free your mind from inner chatter

Bhramari, the humming breath, encourages a long detoxifying out-breath, and purifies and stimulates the throat (vishuddha) chakra (see page 19). It cleanses the mind of "chatter" and clears away self-doubt and the need to gossip, preparing you to discover your unique inner voice and become better able to measure your words. With regular practice, you may find yourself developing the ability to listen more deeply and communicate with others on a more profound level. The joy many people experience from practising this breathing exercise is indescribable – it brings an awareness of great inner peace.

This is highly recommended as a cleansing practice if you are a singer, actor, teacher or public speaker – or for anyone who would like to speak with a purer sounding or more melodious voice and improve their communication skills. With regular practice, it also improves concentration, memory and confidence, and helps to improve throat problems, hoarseness or a weak voice. When you first begin to practise, be aware that you may feel a slight increase in body warmth, as your blood circulation quickens.

Enhance the cleansing effects of Bee Breath by practising it using Shanmukhi Mudra (see opposite), which increases your sensitivity to the physical vibration of sounds.

1 Sit comfortably with your back straight (see pages 24–25); make sure your abdomen and chest are relaxed and open. Rest your palms on your thighs.

2 With lips gently sealed, bring your awareness to the back of the soft palate in the roof of your mouth; slightly tighten the back of your throat. Keep your neck muscles relaxed.

3 Inhale strongly through both nostrils, vibrating your soft palate to make a snoring sound that energizes your throat. Think of it as the sound you make when clearing your throat. Yoga texts liken it to the buzzing of a large black bumblebee or male bee.

4 When ready, exhale through both nostrils, making a high-pitched humming "mmmm" sound. Yoga texts compare this sound to the buzzing of a small honey bee, or a female bee. Try to exhale completely.

5 Repeat 2–3 times. Experiment with different pitches, becoming aware of how the vibration feels in your throat, mouth, cheeks and lips. Notice how humming as you breathe out helps regulate your breath and lengthens your exhalation.

6 Then close your eyes and breathe silently. Sit quietly for 3–10 minutes noticing the effect the humming has had on your mind.

PRACTICE TIPS

- If you find the exercise tricky, begin by practising the humming exhalation only.
- Inhale deeply and repeat a word that ends with an "m" sound, such as "palm", "calm", "hum" or "OM". Draw out the final "m" sound for as long as you can.

> "Inhale the air rapidly, making the sound of a male bee, practise retention and again exhale it, making the sound of a female bee humming. The great yogis by a constant practice of this feel an indescribable joy in their hearts. This is Bhramari." *Hatha Yoga Pradipika*, 2.68

SHANMUKHI MUDRA

This hand gesture is an especially helpful addition to Bee Breath if you have an overly active mind and would like to develop a meditation practice.

1 Sit in a comfortable meditation position with your spine straight and head erect (see pages 24–25). Close your eyes. Insert the tip of each thumb into one of your ears.

2 Lightly touch each closed eyelid with one of your index fingers.

3 Use your middle fingers to apply gentle pressure either side of the bridge of your nose.

4 Rest your ring fingers on your upper lip. Press your little fingers just below your lower lip and gently squeeze your lips closed.

5 Hold this hand position as you practise Bee Breath, trying to keep your face and jaw muscles relaxed and your back teeth slightly separated.

SIMPLE VARIATION

Insert the tip of one thumb into each ear. Fold the other fingers gently into your palms – or simply cup your hands over your ears. Close your eyes as you inhale silently and exhale the humming breath.

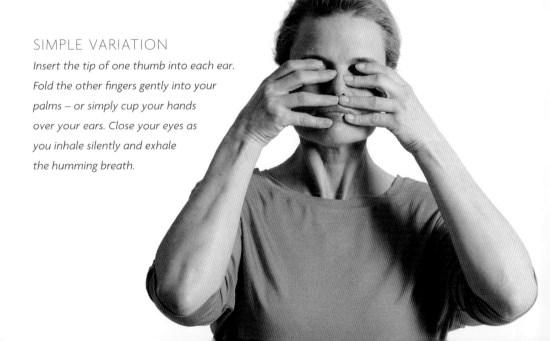

LION'S YAWN POSE: SIMHA KRIYA
To cleanse the throat area

Also known as Simhasana, this ferocious-looking yoga pose is a useful tool for cleansing and revitalizing the throat, face and eyes. In fact it tones the entire cervical-spine region above the shoulders, including the larynx, tonsils, salivary glands, tongue, thyroid and parathyroid. It also cleanses the respiratory system and is said to help prevent laryngitis and other ailments of the throat. The pose is thought particularly beneficial when practised in the early morning facing the rising sun.

This makes an excellent cleansing practice for singers, lecturers, teachers and anyone who engages in public speaking. The cleansing action helps remove blocks to communication and counters reticence, empowering practitioners to feel less restrained and able to express thoughts succinctly.

1 Kneel with your left heel beneath your right buttock and right heel beneath your left buttock. If this is uncomfortable, bring your knees and inner ankle bones together and sit on your heels (a yoga pose known as Vajrasana). Rest your hands on your thighs, palms facing down.

2 Inhale deeply. To exhale, open your mouth wide, stick out your tongue as far as possible and release the air forcefully, making an elongated "Ahhhhhhh" sound. Simultaneously spring forward like a lion poised for attack: straighten your arms, stiffen your body and stretch your fingers to form "claws". Bulge your eyes and direct your gaze to the point between your eyebrows (see Bhrumadhya Drishti, page 46). Hold with the breath out for as long as is comfortable.

3 Sit back on your heels, relax and take a few regular breaths in and out. Repeat 2–5 times.

VARIATION: FOR EXTRA CLEANSING

To stimulate a stronger cleansing of the throat, after you exhale keep your tongue out and then move it from side to side.

SHOULDERSTAND: SARVANGASANA
To remove creative blocks

One of yoga's most important detoxification poses, this inversion acts on the whole body. It helps to drain stagnating blood and lymph caused by the downward pull of gravity while energizing the thyroid, which controls all metabolic processes and regulates the rate at which cells utilize food and oxygen. Regular practice enhances the profound effect of this endocrine gland on physical, emotional and mental wellbeing.

When you perfect Shoulderstand your chin rests on your breastbone, which cleanses the throat and cervical spine. On an energetic level, the pose releases impurities from the throat (vishuddha) chakra (see page 19) and clears communication difficulties such as writer's block

Caution: During pregnancy, practise the Half-shoulderstand variation, below.

1 Place padding under your shoulders, if desired. Lie on your back with your legs extended and together.

2 Bringing your hands to your buttocks, slowly lift your legs and trunk and walk your hands down your back, toward your shoulders. Try to lift yourself as straight as possible, hands flat on your back, fingers pointing toward your spine.

3 Keeping your legs straight, relax your calves and feet. Your chin should press against your breastbone. Soften your face, tongue and throat. (See picture, below right.)

4 If you are a beginner, hold for no longer than 10 seconds. Once comfortable in the pose, gradually increase to 3 minutes.

5 To come down, lower your legs halfway to the ground behind your head; take your hands and forearms to the floor behind your back. Keeping your head down, slowly unroll, lowering the vertebrae one by one.

VARIATION: HALF-SHOULDERSTAND

If the full pose feels too challenging, do not attempt to straighten your body in step 2. Instead, leave legs at an angle (see picture, below left). This pose, Viparita Karani, is recommended by the yoga texts as the best method of reversing the ageing process. It also drains varicose veins and helps to eliminate insomnia.

NECK EXERCISES
To clear away tension

Cleanse your hearing on the concrete physical level by freeing movement in the neck and clearing tension that blocks healthy circulation. These daily exercises also counteract the effects of spending hours with head dropped forward and shoulders hunched (on computers, phones and tablets), which strains the neck and upper-back muscles and can reduce the natural curve of the cervical spine (between neck and skull).

UP AND DOWN
1 Gently nod your head 5–10 times, as if saying "yes".
2 Turn your head 45 degrees to the right and continue nodding. Turn to look over your right shoulder, nodding. Return your head to centre and repeat to the left.

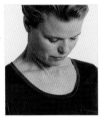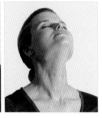

FORWARD AND BACK
1 Keeping your back straight, drop your head to your chest, chin touching your breastbone. Relax; letting the weight of your head release tension in the neck. Hold for 2–3 breaths.
2 Lift your chin as high as you can; let your head drop back. Visualize the back of your head touching your spine. Bring the tips of your front teeth and lips together; take 2–3 breaths.
3 Repeat 3–4 times. The last time you take your head back, open your mouth wide and yawn deeply to release neck tension. Or purse your lips and give the ceiling 4–5 exaggerated juicy kisses. Return your head to its central upright position.

TWISTING FROM SIDE TO SIDE
1 Placing your right hand on your left knee, twist as far to the left as you can. Look over your shoulder. Keep your spine perpendicular.
2 Without moving your shoulders, turn your head right, as if looking behind your back; then look over your left shoulder. Repeat 3–4 times left and right. Come back to centre.
3 With left hand on right knee, repeat on the other side.

CRESCENT MOONS

Without hunching, bring your chin toward the v-shaped point between your collarbones. Move your chin left and right in a gentle crescent 2–3 times. Return the head to centre.

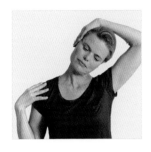

SIDE TO SIDE

1 Bring your left ear toward your left shoulder; don't twist your neck or let your shoulders rise. Hold for 2–3 breaths, then repeat to the right. Repeat 2–3 times in each direction.
2 Take your head to the left, bring your left hand overhead and place your palm over your top ear. Hold for a gentle stretch. Repeat to the right, then return the head to centre.
3 Place the fingers of your right-hand on your right shoulder and drop your head to the left. Bring your left hand overhead to hold your ear; let your hands gently stretch your neck in opposite directions. Bring your head back to centre; repeat on the other side.

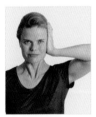
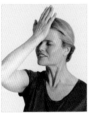

NECK STRENGTHENING

1 Sitting up straight, head directly above your ribcage, place your left palm flat against the left side of your head. Push with your hand and resist with your head for 2–3 breaths (your head won't move), then repeat on the right.
2 Place one palm flat against your forehead. Push back with your hand as your head resists for 2–3 breaths. Drop your hand and take a deep breath.
3 Interlace your fingers and bring them behind your head. Push forward with your hands as your head resists for 2–3 breaths.

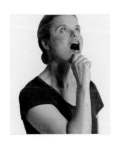

RELEASING TENSION IN THE JAW

1 Hold your lower jaw stationary. Open your mouth by lifting the upper jaw; notice your head tilting back. Repeat 2–3 times.
2 Still holding your chin, lift your upper jaw and roll the skull left and right making miniscule movements; let tension go in the jaw and top of the spine.

SEEKING PURITY OF SPEECH
To detox from judgement and stress

Adhering to the truth – known as *satya* in Sanskrit – is one of the basic tenets of yoga. It is about making a conscious effort to speak the truth and make sure your words as well as your thoughts and deeds are clean, authentic and respectful. This purifies the mind, strengthens inner resolve and attracts positive energy. Expressing feelings in a negative way – even if we don't mean the words we say – tends to draw us away from this state of inner peace and activates distressing energy that flows to the heart (anahata) and brow (ajna) chakras (see page 19) and out into the environment.

The way we speak creates vibrations that not only affect us but everyone we come in contact with – so cultivating purity of speech encourages us to develop a more harmonious relationship with the world around us.

PURIFYING YOUR SPEECH PATTERNS
1 Begin by watching yourself for a few days, just as you are. Try to notice how you speak and interact with other people, being objective and trying not to judge yourself. If you can honestly see your defects, you can begin to overcome them. Decide what you would like to change.

2 Set a practice intention or *sankalpa*: a positive statement that states exactly what you plan to do (there is an example to follow on page 27). Make it definite and determined; commit to an exact technique and amount of practice and avoid vague expressions.

3 Now create an affirmation, a suggestion to repeat to help change your negative speech patterns into more positive ones. Avoid phrases such as "try to, if possible, should" and platitudes, such as "be more peaceful". Use concrete terms and start with "I will". Repeat it consciously, either mentally or out loud.

4 Then just be a silent witness. Notice how, with regular steady practice your language and speech patterns become more positive and compassionate.

> "Purity of speech, of the mind, of the senses, and of a compassionate heart are needed by one who desires to rise to the divine platform."
> Chanakya's *Arthashastra*

VOLUNTARY SILENCE: MOUNA
To retreat and restore

Giving yourself some quiet time each day when you are not distracted by a noisy environment or goal-orientated tasks is a powerful purifying practice known as *Mouna* in the yoga tradition. A few quiet minutes of voluntary silence can prove more relaxing than listening to "relaxing" music. Silence offers your brain the opportunity to let down its sensory guard, process things that have happened during the day, and release physical and mental tension. This has a cleansing restorative effect and helps conserve energy. After Mouna, you may notice increased mental awareness as you go about your everyday life.

Voluntary silence is also about controlling speech when you do talk, refraining from small-talk and the kind of "verbal diarrhoea" that drains us of energy, is distracting and makes it more difficult to focus inward. Watch what happens when you speak less and listen more. You may find, after some time, that you can more easily control your senses and mind. This natural cleansing process of self-analysis helps to bring your words in tune with your actions and thoughts. Then all communication becomes more meaningful.

As you decrease the external noise you make, note the busyness of your internal environment. In the beginning thoughts may arise encouraging you to break your silence: old worries, troubling emotions, an urgent call you need to make. Do not allow yourself to become involved. Watch the thoughts as if they were bubbles, which soon pop or float away. Your anxieties will gradually lessen and it will become easier to remain silent both internally and externally. Once a regular daily silent practice stills your bubbling thoughts and surging emotions, notice how your words have greater power, and you can more easily connect with the inner silence and enjoy a mind that is peaceful and more effective.

PRACTICE TIPS
- Try to observe a period of silence every day – an hour is ideal – or work up to one day of silence each week.
- Practise yoga poses or breathing exercises, walking or simple manual work during your periods of silence.
- Do not listen to music, watch television or read, engage in fast exercise or do anything that requires intellectual focus when silent.
- Try eating one meal a week in full silence; notice the positive effects on your digestion.
- Before speaking "edit" your words. Say only what is required and what is truthful.

CHANTING OM:
NADA-NU-SANDHANA
To invigorate the nervous system

This four-part exercise harnesses the power of the mantra OM to cleanse and energize mind and body. The vibrations set up by the sound of the chanting help transform and energize every part of your body, awakening latent physical and mental powers, but it has an especially positive effect on the nervous system.

The cleansing powers of this exercise derive from two sources: the sound of the mantra and the yogic hand gestures or mudras. The sound OM has no literal translation; it is an abstract sound considered in many ancient yoga texts to be the original vibration by which the universe came into being, and it cleanses your sense of hearing at the highest level (see pages 52–53). In this exercise you break down the sound into its constituent parts A + U + M, and then reintegrate it. When broken into its components, the mantra cleanses not only the cells of the body on a physical level, but affects your being on emotional, mental and subtle levels. The mantra is even more effective when chanted with mudras, which help to channel the vital prana into more positive directions.

THE THREE PARTS OF OM

	A	U	M
Represents	Past	Present	Future
State of consciousness	Waking state	Dream state	Deep sleep
Associated with	Physical plane	Astral / mental plane	Beyond mind and intellect
Sound made with	Mouth wide open	Mouth/lips rounding	Lips shut
Sound vibrates in	Abdomen	Chest	Head and sinuses

Sit in a comfortable meditation position with your spine straight and head erect (see pages 24–25). Do not lie down.

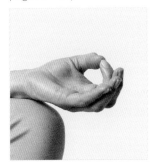

1 Adopt Chin Mudra: join the tips of your thumb and index finger on each hand. Let your other fingers stretch out, but keep them relaxed. Rest the backs of your hands on your thighs. Inhale slowly and completely until your lungs are full. Open your mouth wide and chant the first part of OM – AA – for as long as possible, feeling the sound resonating in your abdomen and the lower parts of your body. Breathe in. Repeat 9 times.

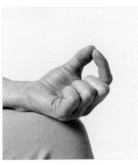

2 Bring your hands into Chinmaya Mudra: join the tips of your thumb and the index finger on each hand. Then fold your middle, ring and little fingers in to touch the palms. Rest the backs of your hands on your thighs. Inhale slowly and completely until your lungs are full. Round your lips and chant the second part of OM – U – for as long as possible, feeling the sound resonating in your chest and the middle part of your body. Breathe in. Repeat 9 times.

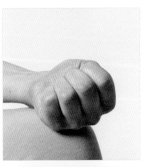

3 Adopt Adi Mudra; fold in your thumbs to touch their respective palms. Then fold the other fingers over the thumb. Rest the backs of your hands on your thighs. Inhale slowly and completely until your lungs are full. Keep your mouth closed and chant the third part of OM – M – for as long as possible, feeling the sound resonating around your head. Breathe in. Repeat 9 times.

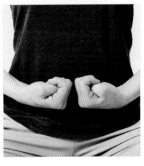

4 Adopt Brahma Mudra: keep your hands in Adi Mudra, but place your fists on either side of your navel. Inhale slowly and completely until your lungs are full. Now repeat all three sounds one after the other: chant AA with your mouth wide open, gradually round your lips to chant U and continue to round your lips until your mouth is closed and you are chanting M. Feel the sound resonating throughout your body. Breathe in. Repeat 9 times.

VICTORIOUS BREATH: UJJAYI
To soothe fear and stimulate the throat

This breathing practice powerfully stimulates and cleanses your throat energy while purifying your hearing as a mental vibration, at its second most concrete level (see pages 52–53). When performed well, Ujjayi creates a soft vibration that soothes the nerves and calms the mind, a great aid to meditation. It also can still fears and is said to counter sadness and depression – the prefix "u" signifies upward expansion. With regular practice, the voice becomes more melodious, and fear of speaking or singing in public vanish. Ujjayi is also said to make you beautiful.

An important exercise in its own right, Ujjayi is often used during yoga posture practice. It cleanses by increasing gastric fire and is valued for clearing excess mucus and coughs, and relieving respiratory problems including asthma, fever and low blood pressure.

HOW IS THE SOUND PRODUCED?

Ujjayi is sometimes referred to as "throat friction". The characteristic sound comes from partially blocking the glottis, the flap at the back of the throat (behind the Adam's apple). The glottis facilitates speech and is the part of the throat that closes when gargling, to prevent water going down your throat.

As you inhale with a partially closed glottis, the slight tension acts as a wind-breaker to incoming air and amplifies the normal sounds of breathing. The friction produces a deep continuous sound. This does not come from the vocal cords, nor is it caused by the friction of air against the soft palate (like in snoring). When doing the exercise well, you will hear a sibilant "sss" sound during inhalation and an aspirant "hhh" during exhalation – if you sound a bit like Darth Vadar you are doing it right!

HOW TO PRACTISE

Remember always to breathe through your nose. If you would like to do more than 20 rounds in one sitting, it is best to practise under the guidance of an experienced teacher.
1 Sit comfortably with your back straight. Close your mouth and inhale slowly through both nostrils, contracting the muscles of your throat near your windpipe to partially close your glottis. Make sure your neck muscles stay relaxed. Listen for a continuous sound at a low but sweet and uniform pitch, similar to a soft sob.

2 At the end of your inhalation, gently pinch both nostrils shut, using your right thumb to close your right nostril, and your ring and little fingers to close your left nostril. Hold your breath for as long as is comfortable.

3 When ready to exhale, release the fingers on your left nostril. Slowly exhale through your left nostril, keeping your right nostril closed with your thumb. This is one round.

4 To begin, practise 5 rounds, always inhaling through both nostrils and exhaling through your left nostril. Gradually build up to 20 rounds in each sitting.

ADVANCED VARIATION WITH MOOLA BANDHA

If you have been practising breathing exercises for a while, you might like to intensify the purifying potential of Ujjayi and other breathing exercises by applying an energetic lock called Moola Bandha during the breath retention. This helps to build a firm physical and energetic foundation for your body and mind.

In men, Moola Bandha results from contracting the muscles around the perineum, midway between the anus and genitals. Women usually feel the contraction more strongly around the base of the cervix. To find which muscles to contract, sit cross-legged with a tennis ball under your perineum. Try to draw your muscles up and away from the ball.

Caution: Avoid Moola Bandha during pregnancy or menstruation, and if you tend toward constipation.

1 While holding your breath in Ujjayi (in step 2), contract your anal sphincter as strongly as possible. Feel as if you are drawing energy up from your pubis, perineum and anus. Use your physical strength to do this, as well as your mental intention and powers of visualization. Draw your pelvic floor toward your chest; imagine your energy moving up along your spine. Visualize all your energies uniting at your heart centre.

2 Release the contraction as you exhale (in step 3).

USING THE BREATH DURING YOGA POSES

Some yoga traditions perform Ujjayi while practising yoga poses. They suggest you keep your glottis partially closed and continue the characteristic sound throughout your practice session. Do not hold your breath; let it come and go continuously at the level of the glottis, trying to keep each inhalation and exhalation at about the same duration. You can also practice Ujjayi while walking.

BATHING THE EARS
To heighten hearing

By freeing the ears of impurities, such as built-up wax, you enhance your powers both of hearing and communication. Ayurveda regards ear problems as a result of vata imbalance – disturbances to the air element (see pages 20–21) that result in itching, wax, issues with balance or ringing in the ears (tinnitus). It suggests we treat vata imbalance with herbal oil.

Caution: Avoid ear washes if you have a problem with your ears.

EVENING HERBAL OIL BATH

Acorus calamus (calamus root), also known as sweet flag, sweet sedge, sweet myrtle or sweet root, is a herb is used by Ayurvedic practitioners to refresh the brain and sharpen memory by promoting circulation. The root is chewed to open the throat chakra and promote inspired speech. Its Sanskrit name *Vacha*, meaning "speech", refers to its effect on the throat chakra and ability to stimulate self-expression and communication. It also enhances meditation.

If you use ginger root in this weekly treatment, pound it in a mortar and pestle and steep in the oil for 30 minutes, then strain. You will need a face cloth and old towel.

1ml (20 drops) calamus oil or 1.5–2cm (½in) fresh ginger root
15ml (3 tsp) organic extra-virgin olive oil or organic sesame oil (untoasted)

1 Mix the oils together, pour into a sterilized dark glass dropper bottle and refrigerate.
2 In the evening, warm the oil by standing the bottle in warm water for a few minutes. Put the towel on your pillow. Lie on one side; drop a few drops of oil in the top ear canal.
3 Close the ear flap and massage the ear canal by pressing gently on the flap in a circular motion for 1 minute. Stop if you experience pain.
4 Gently massage the ear cartilage for 1 minute between thumb, index and middle fingers.
5 Relax on your side for approximately 10 minutes to allow the oil to be absorbed.
6 Turn onto your back, drain excess oil into the face cloth or a tissue and wipe the inside of your ear. Turn onto your other side and repeat.

CLEANSING WITH SOUND
To bathe the chakras

Bathing the chakras in sound cleanses your hearing at a subtle vibrational level (see pages 52–53), helping disperse the limitations put on your communication by preconceptions, sense impressions, emotions and experiences. You let go of what no longer serves you.

1 Sit in a comfortable meditation position, spine straight and head erect (see pages 24–25). Close your eyes and take a few deep breaths. Visualize your breath becoming longer until you feel you are breathing into all the parts of your body in contact with the ground. Feel as though you are growing roots deep into the earth.

2 Every time you inhale, draw energy up from the earth. As you exhale, release what you do not need – physical toxins, emotional impurities, negative emotions – into the earth.

3 After 8–10 breaths in and out, take one hand behind your back, palm facing toward the sacral region (middle of your lower back), about 5cm (2in) from your body. Inhale deeply. As you exhale, chant the sound "mmm", with lips gently closed. Imagine the sound resonating in and cleansing your sacral (swadhisthana) chakra. Repeat for 3–5 breaths.

4 Move your hand in front of your solar plexus and chant "mmm" again as you exhale, feeling the sound resonate in your solar plexus (manipura) chakra. Repeat 3–5 times.

5 Slide your hand up, palm facing your heart. Inhale deeply and chant "mmm" on the out-breath; feel the sound resonate in your heart (anahata) chakra. Repeat 3–5 times.

6 Bring your hand in front of your throat. Chant "mmm" as you exhale, feeling the sound in your throat (vishuddha) chakra. Repeat 3–5 times.

7 Bring your hand in front of your forehead and chant "mmm" on the out-breath; feel the sound resonate in your sinuses and brow (ajna) chakra. Repeat 3–5 times.

8 Raise your hand and hold it over your head, palm down. Chant "mmm" on the exhalation; feel the sound at your crown (sahasrara) chakra. Repeat 3–5 times.

10 Sit quietly for a few minutes, enjoying the cleansing experience of profound silence.

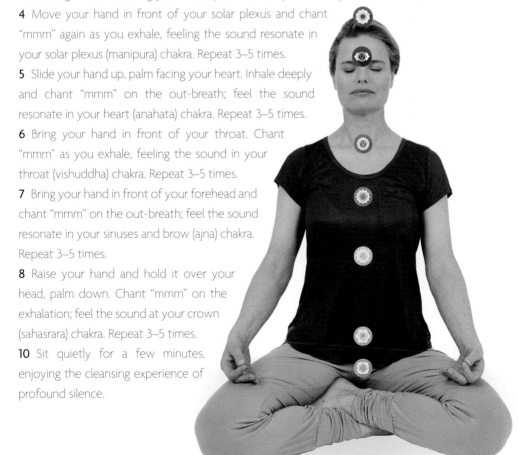

CLEARING THE THROAT: VISHUDDHA CHAKRA MEDITATION
To encourage positive communication

The literal translation of the Sanskrit word *vishuddha*, the throat chakra (see pages 18–19) relates to space as being the purest of elements. When this chakra is cleansed and functioning well you are able to implement decisions, speak up for what you believe in and establish personal boundaries. If your throat chakra is blocked, you may have difficulty in expressing yourself honestly, experience shyness, have difficulty in articulating your feelings, be prone to gossip, fail to keep promises or use words to hurt others. Releasing any blockages enables positive communication but also the healthy flow of your creative energy, since this chakra governs all the faculties involved in self-expression and artistic creativity too: the throat, mouth, tongue and ears. We can cleanse the chakra with affirmations and listening meditations focused on the sound of the breath.

AFFIRMATIONS TO CLEANSE THE THROAT CHAKRA
Sit with your eyes closed and mentally repeat one or more of the following positive statements with full concentration and acceptance:
- I receive intuitive guidance and have the courage to act on it.
- My creative instincts are sound and pure.
- I always speak the truth. My word is my bond.
- My relationships with others are honest and straightforward.
- I communicate my feelings and emotions in healthy ways.
- I strive to understand, as well as to be understood.

SO HAM MEDITATION
In this cleansing meditation you listen to the sound of your breath. On the out-breath it makes the sound "Ham", the mantra of the throat chakra. When practised with Akasha Mudra (see below) you cleanse by freeing up space in your body and mind. Don't worry if at first you can't sit comfortably for 20–30 minutes; build up to it gradually.
1 Sit in a comfortable meditation position, preferably cross-legged, with your spine straight and head erect (see pages 24–25). Rest the backs of your hands on your thighs. Join the tip

of each thumb with the middle finger of the same hand. This makes Akasha Mudra.

2 Suggest to yourself that you will sit still and be fully focused for the next 20–30 minutes. Try not to move a muscle to prevent your mind from being drawn outward.

3 Close your eyes and bring your awareness to your breath. Take 3–4 deep breaths and then let go. Don't try to control your breath, instead concentrate on listening to the natural sound of your breath moving in and out.

4 As you inhale, listen to your breath; hear it repeating the sound "So". Feel your breath joyously drawing in life.

5 As you exhale, hear your breath repeating the sound "Ham". Let go of pent-up tension and aggression. Let go of expectation. Be still and open to the experience.

6 Repeat, fixing your attention on the sound of your breath. Don't try to say the mantras, but listen to your breath as it naturally says them. Gradually your mind will calm. Whenever your mind drifts off, keep bringing it back to your breath.

WHISPERING "AH"

This simple exercise enhances your openness to living a joyous life. It instills a positive state of mental wellbeing that equips you to approach things with a fresh mind. Your thoughts become steady and peaceful and you are better able to be entirely present in the moment.

1 Sit in a comfortable meditation position with your spine straight and head erect (see pages 24–25). Let your tongue rest on the floor of your mouth with the tip lightly touching your lower front teeth. This facilitates the free passage of air at the back of your throat. Breathe gently through both nostrils without attempting to control your breath.

2 Close your eyes and think of something that makes you smile – maybe remember a pleasant experience or think of a friend or a child. This mental act causes you to lift your soft palate, helping to create an even freer flow of air – it also helps release tension from the lips, jaw and facial muscles.

3 Gently, relax your jaw. Keep your lips gently touching, but let your lower jaw drop. Let your teeth come slightly apart; but don't tilt your head back.

4 Inhale, visualizing your breath travelling in horizontally through your nasal passages.

5 Exhale and, keeping your lips as close as possible, softly whisper "ah" until your breath comes to its natural end.

6 Repeat several times; do not rush or force the air out; don't try to extend your breath, but notice how your posture improves and your jaw relaxes.

7 You may like to repeat the exercise whispering: "ee", "oo" and "sss".

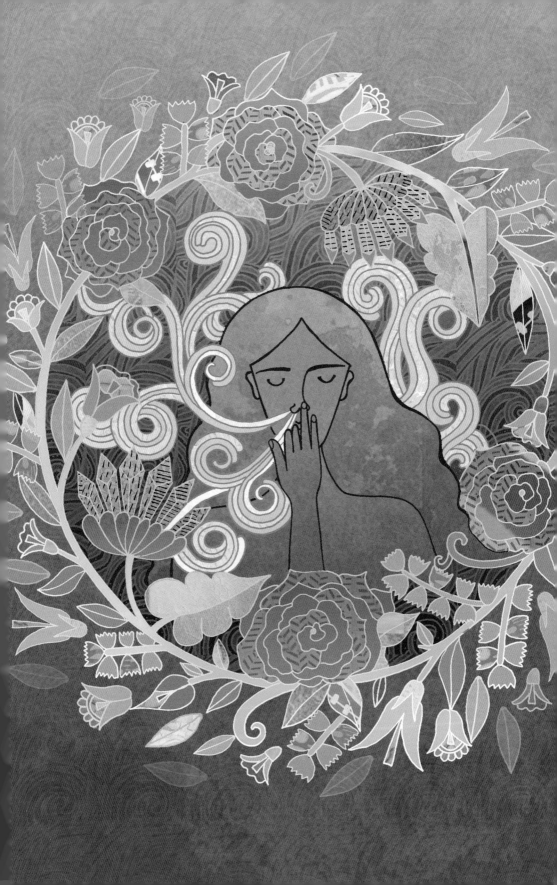

3
BREATHING MORE DEEPLY

TO OPTIMIZE YOUR ENERGY AND SMELL THE ROSES

"A bit of fragrance always clings to the hand that gives roses."
Confucius

"When all the nadis (meridians) that are now full of impurities become purified, then only can the yogi successfully perform pranayama."
Hatha Yoga Pradipika, 2.5

MAXIMIZING YOUR SENSE OF SMELL – AND ENJOYMENT OF LIFE

Yoga puts especially great emphasis on purifying the respiratory system, the body structure that begins with the nose and relates to your sense of smell. This chapter offers cleansing techniques including breathing exercises that encourage stronger lungs, clearer skin and a calmer, more transparent and steady mind. After practising the exercises here you will feel more balanced and energized, and have an increased sense of freedom and joy.

THE SENSE OF SMELL IN YOGA

Smell is the most primitive of your five senses. At the back of each nostril is the olfactory nerve, the shortest major nerve in your body, connecting directly to the brain. This is the nerve that enables you to smell things; it is also the nerve that is stimulated in yoga breathing exercises, known as pranayama.

EFFECTS OF CLEANSING YOUR OLFACTORY ORGANS

Removing obstructions to easy breathing immediately makes a pranayama practice more effective. Start by freeing your airways with Neti followed by Kapalabhati (see pages 74–77). Nasya (see pages 84–85) is a slightly stronger way to clear the upper breathing mechanism and sinuses.

Stimulating pressure points on your face during an Ayurvedic face massage (see pages 86–87) increases blood supply to the facial muscles while helping clear the nasal passages and sinuses. Performed gently, it is one of most effective self-care cleansing techniques and especially beneficial if you spend hours on a computer as it relieves tension and enhances memory. It's a useful preliminary to respiratory steams (see page 117).

On page 79 you will find a technique for checking airflow through your nostrils to assess which one is dominant at any time of day. Having worked this out, you can practise *swara yoga*: observing which nostril has a stronger exhalation and acting accordingly. For example, to do accounts, memorize a poem or plan a party, you would be most efficient breathing predominantly through your right nostril. The connected rational, analytical and mathematical left hemisphere of the brain processes information sequentially, linearly and logically, and is stimulated and cleansed by Sagarbha (see page 82). Conversely, the right hemisphere of your brain deals with information in a diffuse, holistic manner that stimulates creative, artistic and musical abilities. It controls your orientation in space and is particularly sensitive to intuitive experiences that may be intangible to your external sense receptors. You can stimulate this portion of the brain through cooling cleansing exercises, such as the Sheetali and Sitkari breaths on page 83.

Alternate Nostril Breathing (see pages 78–79) encourages activity in both hemispheres of the brain to be equalized: stimulating airflow through both nostrils brings them into balance. On the rare occasion that this equilibrium takes place, your awareness tends to be beyond the normal consciousness of time and space. This is the best time to engage in spiritual activity, such as meditation, prayer and expressions of compassion.

SMELL AND YOUR ENERGY BODY

The exercises in this chapter allow you to tune into the rhythms of different energies in the body, helping you acquire, control, store and distribute prana (see page 18). Practising Samanu (see pages 80–81) for example, clears your subtle energy channels of impurities, helping prana circulate more freely. The energy centre that controls your sense of smell is the root (muladhara) chakra, associated with grounding and letting go. The chapter includes a visualization using mudra hand gestures to cleanse and balance this chakra, leaving you feeling fully present. Balancing your muladhara energy enhances your ability to eliminate what you no longer need or want in life, including negative thoughts and emotions. It can help release you from prejudices and intolerances you may have held for a long time, or negative ways of looking at the world passed on during your early life.

THE FREEDOM OF LETTING GO

By cleansing your sense of smell and root chakra you may find that you can think more clearly, take decisions more decisively and feel better able to take part and savour each moment as it arises – moving through life with an enhanced ability to "smell the roses".

BENEFITS OF CLEANSING YOUR SENSE OF SMELL

• Enhances your perception of both smell and taste.
• Helps you get into "the zone" instantly and be in the moment.
• Enables you to bypass the thinking mind and directly access meditation.
• Strengthens your ability to summon memories instantly.

NASAL CLEANSING: NETI
To free your nasal passages

The nose is designed for purifying the air you breathe. Small hairs filter dust, pollen, pollution and airborne bacteria from the air you inhale, while the shape of the nose brings it to body temperature and humidity before it enters the lungs. If you tend to breathe through your mouth, perhaps because your nose is blocked, you miss out on this protective cleansing and may be susceptible to dry or sore throats and airborne bugs.

Neti is one the six classical yoga cleansing exercises or kriyas (see page 15) and is traditionally used in India as a method of cleansing the nasal passages and sinus cavities, to keep them functioning well and clear from dust, pollen, bacteria and excess mucus. The practice is recommended for everyone, especially people with asthma, allergies and respiratory problems and is easy to pick up. Even if you are not ready to try the method, it is worth knowing about the principles.

THE CLEANSING POWER OF SALTWATER

Neti uses a saline solution. Salt has been used for thousands of years as a natural antiseptic and anti-inflammatory substance. Use natural sea salt, not table salt, which contains chemical additives. Fine sea salt is preferable to coarse because it dissolves more easily. You can use filtered, boiled or bottled water for cleansing the nasal passages, depending on the water in your area; practise Neti with the water you drink. The water can be room temperature or heated a little, if you prefer. Avoid cold water, as it will be uncomfortable.

BATHING THE NASAL PASSAGES: JALA NETI

Practise in the morning after brushing your teeth (twice a day if you feel a cold coming on). You will need a small "neti pot" with spout, from a health store, pharmacy or online, and some fine sea salt.

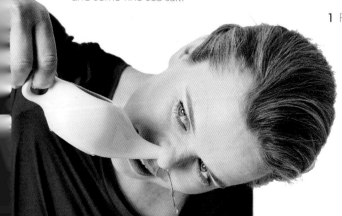

1 Fill the neti pot with the lukewarm water. Add ½ tsp of salt and stir until absorbed. To taste for the right level of saltiness, check that it tastes like tears, not seawater.

2 Leaning over a sink, close the back of your throat (as if about to gargle). Tilt your head to the left and, using the spout, pour the saltwater into your right nostril. Allow gravity to drain the water out through your left nostril. Do not inhale.

3 Blow your nose, then repeat the procedure by tilting your head to the right and pouring the water through your left nostril. Again, do not inhale.

4 When you have cleansed both sides, dry your nasal passages well. Stand with feet well apart and knees slightly bent. Let your head hang down to drain excess water. If you have high blood pressure or feel dizzy, try Alternate Nostril Breathing instead (see pages 78–79).

INTERMEDIATE VARIATION
If you're used to working with the neti pot, you may want to tilt your head back as you pour the saltwater into your nostrils. Spit out the water through your mouth, being careful not to inhale any.

CLEANSING WITH THREAD: SUTRA NETI

This technique, which can seem a little strange to some at first, is best learned with an experienced teacher. At first, you might like to practise it in front of a mirror. Once you are used to it, you may want to practise it up to once a week. You will need 30–45cm (12–15in) cotton cord dipped in beeswax or 3mm red rubber catheter, available online.

Caution: Avoid if you suffer with nose bleeds, nasal ulcers, polyps or have a deviated septum.

1 After Jala Neti, immerse the thread or catheter in the saline solution.

2 Insert the pointed end into one nostril and wiggle. Gently push into the nasal passage.

3 When you feel it in the back of your throat reach your thumb and index finger into your mouth. Then very slowly and carefully pull the thread out through your mouth.

4 Once the thread is completely out, blow your nose and repeat on the other nostril. Dry your nasal passages as in Step 4 of the previous exercise.

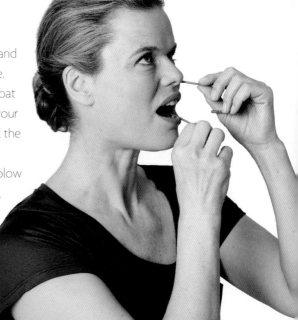

PURIFYING BREATH: KAPALABHATI
To cleanse your respiratory system

Kapalabhati is another of the six classical yoga cleansing exercises or kriyas (see page 15). It purifies your entire system, working primarily on cleansing the respiratory system while strengthening and increasing your lung capacity. The name comes from the Sanskrit words *kapala* meaning "skull" and *bhati* "shining". It is sometimes referred to as *bhalabhati* or "shining forehead" – with regular practice, Kapalabhati is said to purify your entire system so thoroughly that your face starts to shine with vibrant good health and inner radiance.

Physically, the technique works by draining the sinuses and helping to eliminate accumulated mucus. The forced exhalation rids the lungs of stale air, making way for a fresh intake of oxygen-rich air, equipping your red-blood cells to transport good amounts of oxygen and aiding in the general renewal of all body tissues, making it a good practice before other breathing exercises

Kapalabhati also refreshes and invigorates the mind. When practised in the morning, immediately after Neti (see pages 74–75), the subsequent feeling of exhilaration, improved concentration and increased mental clarity often lasts all day.

Caution: Avoid during pregnancy and menstruation or if you suffer from high blood pressure.

PRELIMINARY EXPERIMENT

Before attempting Kapalabhati, sit with your back straight and place your left hand on your abdomen. Raise your right hand approximately 15cm (5in) in front of your mouth; make a gentle fist, thumb pointing upward. Imagine your thumb is a lit candle. Quickly blow out the candle, noticing how your abdomen automatically pulls in with the sharp exhalation. Repeat 5–10 times, imagining that the candle keeps relighting, but this time keep your mouth closed and exhale through your nose. This is a simplified form of Kapalabhati.

TO PRACTISE KAPALABHATI

When you start practising the technique, notice that the technique is exactly the same as in the preliminary exercise where you blew out the imaginary candle. If you feel light-headed you are not doing the exercise correctly. Consult an experienced teacher.

1 Sit in a comfortable meditation position, preferably cross-legged, spine straight and head erect (see pages 24–25). Take 2–3 deep breaths in and out through your nose. Then inhale and begin rhythmic abdominal pumping as follows:

2 Exhale as you contract your abdominal muscles quickly. This causes your diaphragm to move up into your thoracic cavity (see picture, right top), emptying stale air from your lungs and forcefully pushing it out through your nostrils.

3 Relax your abdominal muscles, allowing inhalation to take place automatically (see picture, right middle). Let the in-breath be passive and silent.

4 Exhale again – make it brief, active and audible. Then relax your lungs and allow them to fill with fresh air. Repeat this pumping 20–25 times.

5 End on an exhalation, then take 2–3 deep breaths to return your breathing to normal. This is one round of Kapalabhati.

6 Repeat 2–3 rounds, increasing to 30–50 pumpings per round.

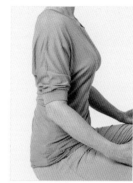

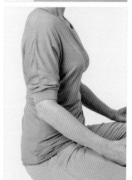

VARIATION: ALTERNATE-NOSTRIL KAPALABHATI – VATA-KRAMA

Once you have mastered Kapalabhati, try this variation which is even more purifying and corrects kapha imbalances (see pages 20–21) that can cause mucus.

1 Raise your right hand and fold the two fingers beside the thumb into your palm (see picture, right bottom). This is known as Vishnu Mudra. You will use the thumb to close your right nostril and your ring and little fingers to close your left nostril.

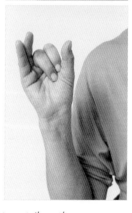

2 Begin Kapalabhati as usual. After 5–10 pumpings, close your right nostril on the exhalation using the thumb of your right hand. On the next exhalation close your left nostril with the ring and little fingers of your right hand. Continue alternating nostrils in this way so you exhale first through one and then the other nostril for approximately 30 pumpings. Don't hold your breath.

3 End on an exhalation and then take 2–3 deep breaths in and out to bring your breathing back to normal. This is one round. Do 2–3 rounds in total.

ALTERNATE-NOSTRIL BREATHING: ANULOMA VILOMA PRANAYAMA
To balance and build energy

Sometimes referred to as Nadi Shoodana Pranayama (cleansing the meridians), this purifying breathing exercise brings the body's two major subtle-energy channels, the ida and pingala nadis, into harmony (see page 18).

When these energy channels fall out of balance, vital energy diminishes. Cleansing them with alternate-nostril breathing restores the balance, equalizing the flow of breath through both nostrils and bringing vigour to body and mind. It also helps to calm the emotions, releases stress and prepares you for meditation. With regular practice, you may notice that you feel much more grounded.

Caution: If practising while pregnant, follow the steps, but do not hold your breath.

1 Sit in a comfortable position; bring your right hand into Vishnu Mudra position by folding your index and middle fingers into the palm of your hand. Do not use your other hand, even if you are left-handed. Raise your right hand in front of your nose, palm inwards.

2 Close your right nostril by pressing with your thumb, and breathe in through your left nostril for a count of 4 (see picture, below left).

3 Gently pinch both nostrils shut and hold your breath for a count of 16 (4 times as long as your inhalation) (see picture, below middle). At the start you may need to hold for just 8 seconds and increase the time gradually.

4 Release your thumb and breathe out through your right nostril for a count of 8 (twice the count of the inhalation) (see picture, below right), keeping your left nostril closed.

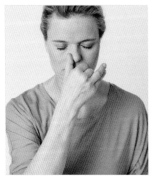 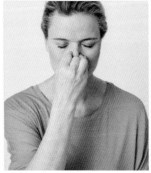 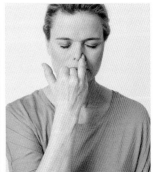

5 Keeping your left nostril closed, breathe in through your right nostril for a count of 4.

6 Close both nostrils and hold your breath for a count of 16.

7 Release your ring and little fingers and breathe out through your left nostril for a count of 8, keeping the right nostril closed. This completes one full round.

8 Aim for at least 10 rounds in one sitting, gradually increasing the number of rounds. As you become more advanced in the practice, you may increase the count, but always keep to the same ratio: 1–4–2. This means that for every second you inhale, retain your breath for four times as long and exhale for twice as long. Never change this ratio.

CLEANSING RIGHT AND LEFT

As explored on page 18, the two main subtle-energy channels or nadis through which the subtle energy yogis know as prana travels are known as ida (on the left) and pingala (right). The right side of your body (controlled by the left side of the brain) is seen as masculine, rational, mathematical, sequential, warm and outwardly directed. It is represented by the Hindu god Siva in the yoga tradition and the yang principle in the Chinese tradition. The left side of the body (right side of the brain) is considered the seat of feminine qualities, as intuitive, simultaneous, cool and inwardly directed. This is represented by the Hindu goddess Shakti, or the Chinese yin principle. When the channels are clear and these principles are in balance our vital energy is strong and we feel calm and grounded.

TO CHECK YOUR BREATH

Try the following experiment, which helps you check which nostril (and energy channel) is dominant at any time of day. The right nostril, referred to as the sun, is the heating channel and represented by the syllable *ha*. The left, symbolized by the moon, is considered cooling and represented by *tha*. The union of the two is referred to as "hatha yoga". Hold a hand beneath one nostril and exhale. Move your hand under the other nostril and exhale. You may notice that your breath is stronger on one side than the other. Repeat the check hourly, noting the dominant side. If you are healthy and don't have a blocked nose your dominant breath will probably change sides every 1½ –2 hours. If you notice your breath flowing equally through both nostrils (quite rare) this as a good time to engage in spiritual activities, such as meditation, prayer and active expressions of compassion. On these occasions your awareness is said to be "beyond time and space".

CLEARING THE ENERGY CHANNELS: SAMANU
To encourage optimal energy flow

In order for the subtle energy known as prana to circulate freely through the energy channels or nadis (see page 18) they need to be free from blockages. You can purify them by physical means, such as with Neti (see pages 74–75) or Alternate Nostril Breathing (see pages 78–79). But you can also do it mentally using the exercise below, known as Samanu, which literally translates from the Sanskrit as "with mind". This cleansing technique combines Alternate Nostril Breathing with chanting various *bija* (seed) mantras – of the elements air, fire and earth – and visualizing key chakras being cleansed of impurities.

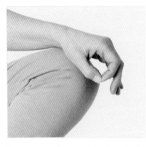

STARTING POSITION
1 Sit in a comfortable meditation position, preferably cross-legged with your spine straight and head erect (see pages 24–25).
2 Join the tips of the thumb and index finger on your left hand. Rest the inside wrist of your left hand on your left knee, fingers pointing downward. This hand position, known as Jnana Mudra, helps to steady your mind and ground your energy.
3 Raise your right hand and fold the two fingers beside the thumb into your palm. This is known as Vishnu Mudra (see page 78). You will use the thumb to close your right nostril and your ring and little fingers to close your left nostril.

AIR PURIFICATION
1 With your hand still in Vishnu Mudra, close your right nostril with your right thumb. Inhale through your left nostril, mentally repeating the mantra of air, YAM. Inhale until you have filled your lungs. As you do this, fix your attention on your heart (anahata) chakra, the energy centre associated with the air element. Visualize air or wind, which is smokey-coloured, flowing through the nadi energy channels in your body, blowing away impurities.
2 As you finish the inhalation, gently pinch both nostrils closed. Hold your breath, keeping your focus on your heart chakra as you continue to mentally repeat the mantra YAM.

3 Release the thumb from your right nostril. Exhale very slowly through your right nostril as you mentally repeat YAM. Let your attention remain on your heart chakra.

FIRE PURIFICATION

4 Inhale through your right nostril, mentally repeating RAM, the mantra of fire. As you do so, fix your attention on your solar plexus (manipura) chakra just below the sternum. Visualize fire burning away all psychic, emotional and mental impurities.

5 Close both nostrils and hold your breath as you mentally repeat RAM.

6 Release your left nostril. Exhale slowly through the left as you repeat RAM mentally. Keep your focus on your solar plexus chakra.

WASHING AWAY IMPURITIES WITH DIVINE NECTAR

7 Inhale through your left nostril, mentally repeating TAM, mantra of the moon, the minor chakra located just inside your left eyebrow.

8 Close both nostrils and hold your breath while repeating TAM. Imagine divine nectar from the moon centre flowing through your nadis, cleansing and soothing away impurities.

GROUNDING

9 Bring your attention to your root (muladhara) chakra at the base of your body as you exhale very slowly through your right nostril. As you exhale, mentally repeat LAM, the mantra of the earth element. Feel as though this mantra is grounding you.

Repeat this entire sequence (steps 1–9) 1–3 times, then release your nostrils, lower your right hand and bring it into Jnana Mudra on your right knee by bringing the tips of the thumb and index finger together. Place both hands in the same position with fingers pointing downwards and sit silently for at least 10 minutes with your full attention on your root chakra. Continue to mentally repeat the mantra LAM. Feel secure, fully present and aware of your connection with the earth.

CLEANSING WITH MANTRA, COLOUR AND BREATH: SAGARBHA
To enhance your potential

This cleansing technique offers such vast potential that it derives its name from the Sanskrit words *sa* "with" and *garbha* "womb". It cleanses by combining colour visualization and breathing alongside the three constituent sounds that make up the "life-giving" mantra OM (A + U + M), the seed sound thought by many texts to be the source of all other mantras. Sweating while practising is considering a good cleansing sign, indicating that you are performing the exercise successfully. Traditionally perspiration is rubbed back into the body to conserve vital energy, making the body more alert and countering fatigue. But if the sweating feels too much, practise one of the cooling breath techniques opposite.

1 Sit in a comfortable meditation position (see pages 24–25). Try to face north or east to benefit from the earth's magnetic currents. Do not lie down.

2 Start by practising a few rounds of Alternate Nostril Breathing (see pages 78–79), then drop your hand and allow your breath to return to its natural rhythm; let it be as fast or as slow and as deep or as shallow as it wants to be. Just watch your breath.

3 After 3–4 breaths, begin to hear the breath mentally repeating the sound OM on the in-breath and OM again on the out-breath.

4 Now raise your right hand and fold the first two fingers into your palm: Vishnu Mudra.

5 Use your right thumb to close your right nostril. Inhale through your left nostril, mentally repeating the first sound of OM – AA, the primal sound a child makes. Visualize red, the colour of creative energy and *rajas* (movement). Inhale for as long as feels comfortable.

6 At the end of the inhalation, keep the thumb on your right nostril and close the left nostril with your ring and little fingers. With both nostrils closed, hold your breath for as long as is comfortable, mentally repeating the middle sound of OM – U. Visualize dark blue, the colour of balance and the infinite sky.

7 Release your thumb and exhale through your right nostril, mentally repeating the final sound of OM – M – as you visualize the cleansing energy of the colour white.

8 Inhale through your right nostril focusing on the sound AA and the colour red. Pinch both nostrils closed and mentally repeat the sound U as you visualize dark blue. Exhale through your left nostril, hearing the sound M and visualizing the colour white. This is 1 round. Complete 5–10 rounds.

CALMING BREATHS: SHEETALI AND SITKARI PRANAYAMA
To refresh your system

Helping remove impurities from the body, these breathing exercises are said to reduce hunger and thirst while lowering temperature and making the body feel lighter and movement more effortless. Sheetali cools the system and is recommended to ease chronic problems thought in the yoga system to arise from excess heat in the body. These include fever, skin rashes, stomach ulcers and hyperacidity, but also for soothing bee stings and fiery conditions of the mind and emotions – the Sanskrit word *sheetali* can be interpreted to mean "calm", "passionless" and "unemotional". The alternative breath, Sitkari, has many of the same effects. It is also said to enhance the beauty and vigour of your body, developing balance, harmony and one-pointed focus.

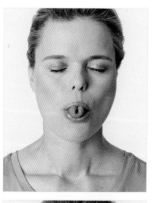

COOLING BREATH: SHEETALI

1 Sit in a comfortable position with your back straight. Stick your tongue out a little way past your lips. If you have the right genes, you will be able to roll the sides of your tongue upward to form a tube. If you can't don't worry; practise Sitkari (below) instead.

2 Draw air into your mouth through your tongue-tube, as though drinking through a straw, making a hissing sound like a snake. Hold your breath for as long as is comfortable, then exhale through both nostrils. Repeat 3–5 times.

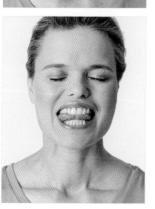

HISSING BREATH: SITKARI

1 Sit in a comfortable position with your back straight. Fold your tongue back so the tip touches the hard ridge behind your teeth. Try to bring your teeth together.

2 Draw air in through your mouth making a hissing sound, "Si-si-si". Then exhale slowly through both nostrils. Repeat 2–3 times.

NASAL OIL CLEANSE: NASYA
To promote clarity of mind

In Ayurveda, the traditional holistic medicine of India, the nose is viewed as the gateway to much more than the respiratory system – it is also the portal to the nervous system, brain and even consciousness itself. Nasya, the administration of herbal-infused oil to the nasal passages, is said to cleanse and strengthen not only the nose, but the eyes, ears, brain, sinuses and throat. It enhances the effects of Neti (see pages 74–75) and pranayama breathing techniques while relieving sinus congestion, eye-strain and clearing the voice-producing mechanisms.

Nasya, also valued for promoting clarity of mind, sharpening the senses and improving sleep patterns, is often prescribed in Ayurvedic medicine to treat mental and emotional imbalance and memory issues, as well as chronic headaches, stiffness in the neck, jaw or shoulders and any imbalances of the doshas that may arise after cleansing treatments (see pages 20–22). Even if you are not ready to try the technique, you might like to find out more about the principles.

Caution: Avoid Nasya during pregnancy, menstruation, after meals and drinking alcohol, when exceptionally thirsty or fasting.

TO MAKE NASYA OIL
Omit the essential oils if you are taking medication for a health condition.

10ml (2 tsp) organic sesame oil (untoasted)

8–10 drops of any of the following combinations of essential oils (preferably organic):

- Eucalyptus and peppermint oils to clear the nasal passages
- Brahmi and sandalwood to calm the mind

Pour the sesame oil into a clean dark glass bottle with a dropper. Add the essential oils, if using, then shake well to combine. Store for future use.

PERFORMING NASAL OIL CLEANSE

You might want to include Nasya as part of your morning cleanse, after brushing your teeth and Neti; it may be practiced at other times of day as well. If you're not used to it, the practice may seem a little strange at first, but it's not uncomfortable. You will need a face cloth and towel.

1 Warm the face cloth and place it over your nose and sinuses. Warm the Nasya oil (see recipe opposite) by standing the bottle in a bowl of warm water.

2 Lie on your back with your limbs extended and feet slightly raised. Roll the towel and place it under your neck so your head tips back slightly.

3 Close one nostril and, using the dropper, place 2–8 drops of oil into the other nostril; sniff it in. Repeat on the opposite nostril, then gently massage around the nose, sinuses and cheeks.

4 Relax in this position allowing the oil to penetrate. After a few minutes, turn onto your side and spit out any oil that may have reached your mouth and throat. Finish by gargling with warm water.

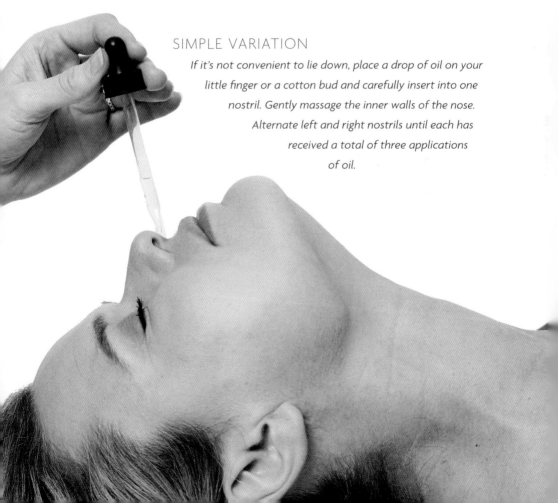

SIMPLE VARIATION

If it's not convenient to lie down, place a drop of oil on your little finger or a cotton bud and carefully insert into one nostril. Gently massage the inner walls of the nose. Alternate left and right nostrils until each has received a total of three applications of oil.

AYURVEDIC FACE MASSAGE
To give you back your glow

This simple self-massage of the face, or facial *abhyanga*, goes more than skin-deep, working on *marma* pressure points energetically linked to the chakras (see pages 18–19). These tiny eye-like subtle-energy centres are located on nadi channels throughout the body, with a quarter thought to be found on the head and face.

When marma points become partly or completely closed as a result of stress, poor diet or injury, the face can appear strained and dull, and there may be an accompanying sense of disconnection or confusion. A cleansing Ayurvedic face massage helps to reopen the marmas, allowing prana to return to the face and leaving it looking more fresh and alive. Then there are the benefits of the massage itself, including the elimination of toxins from increased circulation and lymph flow, glowing skin and the release of tension, which may reduce the appearance of fine lines.

This massage is most effective as part of a morning cleansing routine, after brushing your teeth and practising Neti (see pages 74–75).

Apply ½ teaspoon of massage oil (see opposite) over clean skin, from the collarbones up and out over the face.

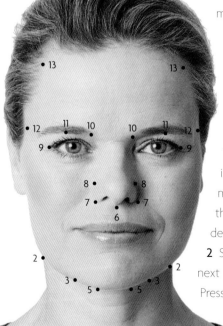

When massaging your face, use your thumbs to make gentle clockwise circles on the points shown on the photograph and outlined in the steps below. Press just enough to feel resistance from the bone or muscle below the skin, circling each point 15–30 times. Release the pressure, but keep your thumb on the skin, and slide to the next point.

1 Start the massage by pressing both thumbs into the marma points where each collarbone meets the breastbone. Release down toward the waist. This helps to boost energy and detox anger.

2 Slide the thumbs up the sides of neck to the next points, 4 finger-widths below the earlobes. Press and circle 15–30 times to improve circulation to the face and stimulate lymphatic drainage.

3 Slide the thumbs inward to each side of the jawbone. Press and massage upward just behind the bone. This improves facial circulation and strengthens the voice.

4 Gently slide the thumbs back down the neck to the V of the clavicle notch. Press gently in a downward direction to clear the voice and upper respiratory congestion.

5 Slide the thumbs up to either side of the centreline of the chin and press. This helps to improve circulation to the face and connects you with your innermost feelings.

6 Press on the point in the middle of the upper lip, to improve mental clarity.

7 Press on the side of each nostril where it joins the face.

8 Press on the points halfway up the nose on either side. This helps clear the sinuses and enhance the benefits of Neti (see page 74) and Nasya (see page 84).

9 Gently massage the outside of each eye to help relieve eye strain.

10 Press the point just above the inside of each eyebrow. Gently press upward, away from the eye to ease eye-strain and headaches.

11 Press the point just above the middle of each eyebrow to feel more centred.

12 Press the point just above the outside of each eyebrow. Then slide your thumbs out to the hollow of each temple; this is said to improve memory.

13 Finally, slide the thumbs up the middle of each half of the forehead. Rub in a gentle clockwise spiral to relieve tension and bring mental peace.

CHOOSING A FACIAL MASSAGE OIL

Try a light, calming oil, such as jojoba. If your skin is particularly dry, add a little rosehip seed and/or avocado oil. For oilier skins, lighter apricot or grapeseed oil is best. Ayurvedic blends include *karpasasthyadi thailam. Karpasa asthi* means cotton seed, its main constituent.

BENEFITS OF CLEANSING FACIAL MASSAGE

• Clears the subtle-energy channels (nadi) in which life-force (prana) flows (see page 18), and stimulates the movement of physical and subtle energy.

• Balances the mix of vata, pitta or kapha energy in your constitution (see pages 20–21).

• Improves sleep, reducing fatigue, restoring the body and boosting immune response.

• Calms the nerves, picks up low spirits and boosts self-confidence.

• Supports all the senses, and helps to relieve eye-strain.

• Improves memory.

• Encourages the clarity and patience you need to make good lifestyle choices.

GROUNDING AND LETTING GO: MULADHARA CHAKRA VISUALIZATION
To help you savour each moment

When the energy of your root (muladhara) chakra (see page 19) is balanced you feel grounded, fully present in the moment and comfortable in your body. There's a sense of being able to live consciously on the earth and draw sustenance from it. This enables you to let go of things you no longer need or want in your life. This cleansing can release physical toxins from your body, and also negative emotions and attachments to relationships that no longer work for you, promoting general good health, and emotional and mental wellbeing.

Try to practise this visualization for at least 10 minutes daily, preferably in the morning before going to work. If you hold the hand gesture Bhu Mudra during the visualization, you create a firm foundation for your practice and encourage unwanted energy to release down into the ground. In Sanskrit, "Bhu" is a name for our planet, Earth.

1 Sit in a comfortable meditation position with your spine straight and head erect (see pages 24–25) – do not lie down. Bring your hands into Jnana Mudra or Bhu Mudra (see opposite). Close your eyes and think about the qualities of earth. Feel as though you are rooting yourself firmly in the present moment, drawing stability and strength up from the ground. Pay particular attention to the pull of gravity and its effects on your body.

2 After a few moments bring your awareness to your breath. Visualize your breath becoming longer until you are breathing into the parts of your body in contact with the ground (or your chair): your buttocks, legs and feet. Imagine yourself growing roots deep into the earth.

3 Continue sitting in this way for at least 10 minutes. Every time you inhale, feel as though you are nurturing yourself by drawing up positive energy (prana) from the ground.

4 With each exhalation, let go of what you no longer need or want to hold onto. The out-breath is the cleansing portion of the breath. If you find it helpful, imagine hearing your breath saying "let go" with each exhalation.

WISDOM GESTURE: JNANA MUDRA

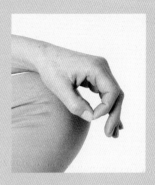

1 Join the tip of each index finger with the thumb of the same hand, forming a circle. You don't need to press hard; just make sure your fingers are making a connection.
2 Gently rest the insides of your wrists on their respective knees or thighs so that your fingers and palms are facing downward. Be careful not to create tension by trying to grab your knees for support.

TOUCHING THE EARTH GESTURE: BHU MUDRA

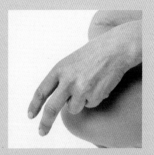

Using both hands, fold your ring and little fingers and your thumb into your palms. Keep your middle and index fingers straight, but relaxed. Rest your hands on your knees, palms facing downward so that your fingers form a downward-pointing and relaxed inverted "V" shape.

THE CLEANSING QUALITIES OF EARTH

In yoga philosophy, "earth" is a term that includes all solid matter; it represents stability, groundedness, being rooted in the present moment and having a firm foundation for life. The earth is the source of all treasure, including the life-giving wealth we all need: food.

If you are the kind of person who spends too much time "in your head" or you tend to feel disconnected, cleansing the muladhara chakra with this visualization can bring great benefit. It is helpful if you are experiencing paralysis, physical or psychological, or feel "stuck" in some way. It helps neutralize the effects of being ungrounded. These include thinking less clearly and having difficulty making decisions. Taken to an extreme, being ungrounded can cause us to detach from the "real" world; we may have problems being on time, be hypersensitive, not listen to what is being said, and have difficulty in following instructions.

If you have spent most of your life being ungrounded, cleansing grounding practices may make you feel a little heavy at first. However, it is well worth persevering; yoga philosophy teaches that when your body is properly grounded you are less likely to absorb the negative effect of toxins physical, emotional and from relationships.

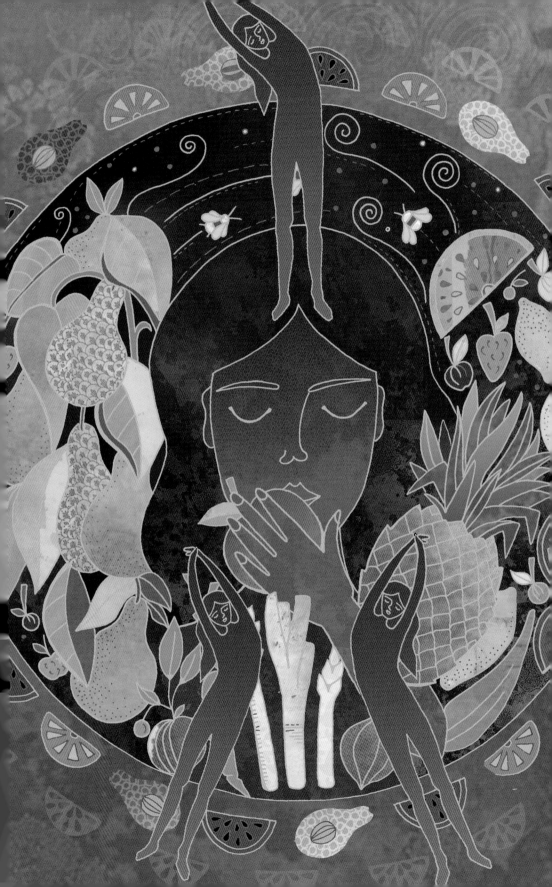

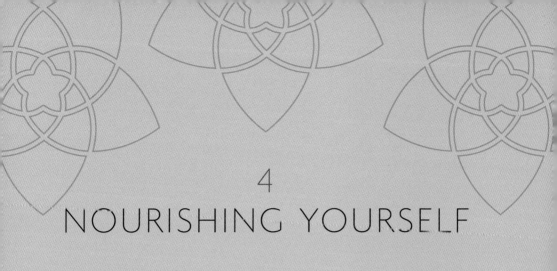

4
NOURISHING YOURSELF

FOR A LIGHTER MIND AND BODY

"Purity of thought depends on purity of food. You can see better, hear better, taste better and think better when you entertain positive, uplifting thoughts."
Swami Sivananda

"The ancient rishis have said that taste has many varieties: sweet, salty, bitter, astringent, sour and acrid. In full there are six sorts of taste, which are thought to be forms of water."
Mahabharata, 12.184.31

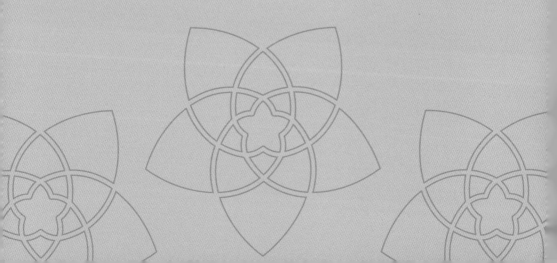

PURIFYING YOUR DIGESTION – TO TASTE ALL LIFE HAS TO OFFER

Yoga teachings encourage you to eat a "pure" diet, rich in fresh vegetables and fruit, wholegrains and legumes, nuts and seeds to increase vitality and build strength and mental clarity. In addition, programmes are recommended to cleanse the digestive system and boost the efficiency of the body's main organ of detoxification, the liver. You will find some in this chapter alongside fasting techniques to give your whole system an overhaul. Fasting has the benefit of lightening the mind and developing patience, willpower and gratitude for the ingredients of life and all there is to taste in the world.

THE SENSE OF TASTE IN YOGA

Yoga philosophy notes that the preferences of your tongue can be an important indicator of your digestive health and your state of wellbeing in general because the experience of eating is often based more on past experiences and life values than on the actual taste of food. Yogic eating – a *sattvic* diet (see pages 98–99) that nourishes and soothes the body while calming the mind and sharpening the intellect – encourages you to eat more consciously and with full focus, becoming aware of taste, texture, aroma and colour and using all your senses to appreciate the food on your plate and in your mouth. Daily tongue cleaning (see page 94) enhances this by stimulating the taste buds.

You are encouraged to stop eating before you feel completely full. The *Hatha Yoga Pradipika* suggests filling the stomach halfway with food, a quarter with liquid and leaving the balance empty to allow digestion the space it needs to take place. Chewing well is also valued in the yoga tradition – Gandhi quotes the American poet Walt Whitman's advice to "drink your solids and chew your liquids". Because digestion begins in the mouth, it is best to chew your food so thoroughly that it becomes liquid. And by "chewing" juices or soups instead of swallowing them down, you enhance your ability to digest them.

EFFECTS OF CLEANSING YOUR DIGESTION

The techniques in this chapter to cleanse the upper digestive tract (Dhauti, see page 107), lower digestive tract (Basti, see page 111) and abdomen (Nauli, see page 109) are considered the foundation of all internal cleansing by the ancient yoga texts. They cleanse the body to ensure optimum functioning and help you pursue your life goals with energy and ease.

It's recommended that you practise some yoga taste-cleansing techniques daily, for example building tongue cleaning and gum massage (see pages 94–95), tongue exercises and oil pulling (see pages 96–97) into your regular tooth-brushing regime.

Other techniques are best practised when winter turns to spring and summer turns into autumn. This includes a 24-hour liver cleanse (see pages 102–103), a yoga sequence to clear the alimentary canal (Shankh-prakshalana, see pages 104–105) and Basti to detox the lower digestive tract (see page 111). These times of year are best for cleaning out waste matter that may have accumulated during the stagnation of the previous months. After bi-annual cleansing your body can begin again, refreshed and renewed. Regular fasting is recommended to rest the digestive system and enhance health and vigour (see page 100–101), whether replacing one meal a week with juice or fruit or doing a fuller seasonal fast, a technique used since ancient times to strengthen the purifying power of meditation.

TASTE AND YOUR ENERGY BODY

As any substance that comes into contact with your tongue must be chewed and mixed with saliva before it can be tasted, yoga philosophy relates the element of water to the sense of taste. Shankh-prakshalana cleanses with water, but other elements can also be used to cleanse this sense. Vata-sara (see page 106) uses air while the Agni-sara exercise (see page 108–109) stimulates your body's "inner fire", invigorating the subtle energy required to digest and absorb not only food but ideas and other essential nourishment.

TASTING MORE KEENLY

Yoga eating encourages you to sit quietly before beginning to eat, take some breaths and think of all you have to be grateful for. You may want to say some words of gratitude – for your food and life in general. Then your sense of taste becomes more than a means of relieving physical hunger and you find ways to get more sweetness in your life.

BENEFITS OF CLEANSING YOUR SENSE OF TASTE

• Increases your preference for healthy foods and helps overcome unhealthy cravings.
• Boosts digestion and absorption of food.
• Strengthens your experience of life's sweetness and ability to embrace all it offers.
• Strengthens your ability to summon memories instantly.

CLEANING THE TEETH, TONGUE AND GUMS
To enhance your sense of taste

Cleaning the mouth is an essential part of a yogi's morning routine. Start with tongue cleaning, then brush your teeth, massage your gums and move on to Oil Pulling and tongue exercises (see pages 96–97). Finally, drink a large glass of water.

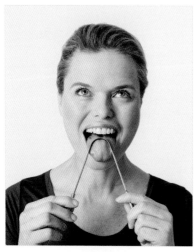

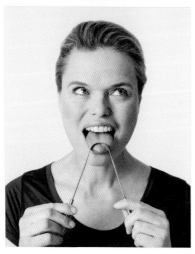

TONGUE CLEANING

This yogic tradition is recommended for clearing unhelpful bacteria from the mouth and promoting healthy gums and good oral health. By removing the coating on the tongue you eliminate a cause of bad breath and enhance your sense of taste by stimulating the taste buds. Practised first thing in the morning tongue cleaning stimulates the entire digestive tract, initiating a cleansing that goes all the way to the lower intestines. Tongue cleaning is said to prevent imbalances of kapha (see page 21) in the form of mucus, which can obstruct effective breathing. Practise daily, first thing in the morning on an empty stomach. You will need a tongue cleaner available from health stores or online.

1 Hold one end of the cleaner in each hand. Extend your tongue (try to relax it). Put the cleaner as far back on the tongue as comfortable.

2 Gently pull the cleaner forward to remove any coating. If this stimulates the natural expelling of mucus and *ama* (toxins) from the back of the throat, spit it out. Rinse the cleaner.

3 Repeat 3–5 times, or until no more coating is removed and your tongue feels clean.

THE CLEANSING POWER OF COPPER

Traditionally, tongue scrapers were made of gold, silver, copper, tin or brass. Today, stainless steel is probably most popular. However, recent research suggests a copper tongue cleaner may be the most cleansing option. Copper has been used for centuries as a bacterial-resistant metal and provides important enzymes that encourage healthy microbes to survive in the mouth.

TOOTH BRUSHING

Ayurveda, the holistic traditional medicine of India, recommends different herbal toothpastes for different constitutional types, whether you have a vata, pitta or kapha dosha (see pages 20–22). This encourages the healthy flow of saliva, essential for cleansing the mouth, stimulating digestion and controlling plaque. Keep the following ingredients in mind when choosing a toothpaste or powder:

Vata-dominant constitutions: Prone to receding gums; choose a toothpaste or powder containing herbs with a bitter-sweet or astringent taste, such as liquorice, cinnamon, fennel, ginger or lemon.

Pitta-dominant constitutions: Prone to bleeding gums; choose a toothpaste or powder containing bitter-tasting herbs, such as neem, bay leaf, benzoin, myrrh or sage.

Kapha-dominant constitutions: Prone to pale gums; choose a toothpaste or powder containing herbs with a pungent taste, such as anise, basil, tulsi (holy basil), caraway, cardamom, cloves, eucalyptus, peppermint and other mints, tea tree or wintergreen.

GUM MASSAGE

Massaging the gums decreases blood stagnation and increases their supply of prana. It leaves the gums feeling really fresh.

1 After brushing your teeth, rinse your mouth with warm water. Wash your hands.

2 Put one thumb into your mouth and with the pad gently massage the gums on the inner and outer parts of the upper and lower jaw using a circular motion for 1 minute.

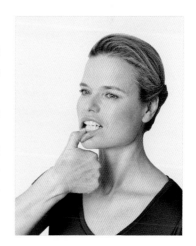

OIL PULLING: KAVAL DHARNAM
To eliminate harmful bacteria

This technique is considered by yogis to be a an effective way to guard against tooth cavities and eradicate bad breath. It helps to eliminate many harmful bacteria in the mouth before they spread to other parts of the body. It is also valued for strengthening the tongue and gums and helping to reduce plaque and plague-induced gingivitis. The essential oils have natural antibiotic and antiviral properties and are recommended by yogis for brighter cleaner teeth. Practise first thing in the morning on an empty stomach, ideally after tongue cleaning (see page 94).

Oil pulling is not a substitute for brushing teeth. Avoid swallowing the oil. If you are pregnant, breastfeeding or taking medication for a health condition, omit the essential oils You will need 30ml (2 tbsp) organic sesame oil (untoasted), coconut or extra-virgin olive oil, plus optional antimicrobial essential oil, such as tea tree, oregano or lemon.

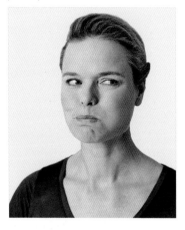

1 Prepare the oil, adding 1 drop only of the antimicrobial essential oil, such as tea tree, oregano or lemon, if preferred; mix well.

2 Place a large spoonful of the oil into your mouth and swish it around for up to 20 minutes as you dress or make the bed, or until your mouth becomes tired.

3 Spit out the oil (not into a sink, which may block the drain), then brush your teeth (see page 95) and rinse your mouth. If possible, follow with tongue exercises (see opposite).

VARIATION: CHEWING CARDAMOM

If you don't have time for Oil Pulling, chew 1–2 cardamom seeds. They make an excellent mouth freshener that promotes oral health by increasing saliva, strengthening the mucosal lining of the digestive system, speeding digestion and reducing heartburn.

TONGUE EXERCISES
To reduce tension

Exercising the tongue is recommended in yoga texts for many health conditions, from insomnia to high blood pressure, facial paralysis, tinnitus and throat infections. Many yogis find that regular practice brings a "fresher" mind, improvements in memory, digestion and absorption of food, and reduced cold and flu symptoms. Practise each morning after washing your face and Oil Pulling (see opposite). If your mouth feels dry, sip water

1 Stand in front of a mirror. Begin by sticking out your tongue as far as possible and moving it back and forth to the far left and right quickly, like a snake. Repeat 10–20 times.

2 Keeping your tongue out, lick your lips clockwise, then anti-clockwise (5–10 times each).

3 Bring your tongue back into your mouth and repeat these circular motions, licking the gums and teeth behind the lips. Repeat 3–10 times clockwise and then anti-clockwise.

4 Draw 10 circles clockwise on the inside of your right cheek, then 10 anti-clockwise. Repeat on the inside of your left cheek.

5 Stick out your tongue as far as you can. Try to bring the tip as close to the tip of your nose as possible – then take it down toward your chin. Repeat up and down 5–10 times.

6 Push your tongue past your lower lip and use it to open your mouth, by pressing down.

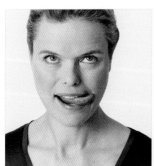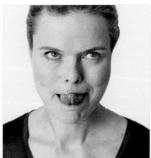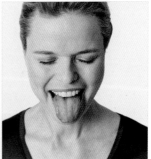

TONGUE TURNING: KHECHARI MUDRA

This is a simple form of one of the most common kriya-yoga cleansing techniques (see pages 14–15). It cleanses and calms the mind, preparing it for meditation.

1 Turn your tongue back so the under surface touches the upper part of the soft palate. Reach the tip of the tongue as far back toward the back of the throat as possible.

2 Hold for as long as is comfortable. Release and relax the tongue, then repeat.

NOURISHING YOURSELF

97

A PURIFYING DIET
To encourage mind-body balance

Eating well, in yogic terms, is about building your diet around *sattvic* foods: pure, wholesome ingredients that are naturally delicious and don't rely on preservatives or artificial flavourings. A sattvic diet is easily digested and supplies maximum energy, helps to eliminate fatigue and powers you through strenuous tasks. And while soothing and nourishing the body it brings calmness to the mind and sharpens the intellect.

Yoga philosophy refers to three qualities that exist in nature: *sattva, rajas*, and *tamas*. They are present in varying proportions in all objects, gross or subtle – including food – and because these qualities operate on physical, mental and emotional levels, they have an effect on your mind, intellect and ego as well as on your body. The quality of sattva is characterized by cheerfulness, peace, contentment and devotion, so building your daily diet around sattvic foods, such as vegetables, wholegrains, nuts and seeds, helps you toward greater purity and self-knowledge.

The quality of rajas, in comparison, manifests in passion and motion, and is associated with over-activity and a restless mind. The mental agitation rajas leads to desire and passions such as anger, envy, greed and jealousy. Rajasic foods, such as processed meals and salty snacks (see chart opposite), are said to arouse "animal passions" and bring about a restless mental state that is unhelpful for inner-peace and lasting happiness. It's best to try to avoid these foods, or enjoy them only occasionally.

The quality of tamas manifests as inertia and laziness. Whereas sattva is associated with purity and knowledge, the quality of tamas is connected with its opposite: darkness and ignorance. So eating tamasic foods, such as meat or overcooked or burnt dishes (see chart opposite), is thought to bring about feelings of dullness or heaviness of mind and make us feel lethargic, lacking in motivation and can aggravate chronic health conditions. Overeating is considered a tamasic activity.

> "My refusing to eat flesh occasioned an inconvenience, and I was frequently chided for my singularity, but with this lighter repast I made the greater progress, from greater clearness of head and quicker comprehension."
> Benjamin Franklin (1706–1790), on his vegetarianism

HOW TO EAT WELL

- Try to eat meals to a regular schedule – and don't snack between meals.
- Eat slowly, chew thoroughly and savour your food. Remember that the digestive process begins in your mouth.
- Sit down to eat and eat in silence, not while working at a computer or checking messages on your phone.
- Try to maintain a peaceful attitude while eating; don't eat when angry or upset.
- Do not overload your stomach; stop eating before you feel full.
- When you have finished eating, sit for a few minutes before leaving the table.
- If you would like to change your diet, introduce new healthy sattvic foods and cut out rajasic and tamasic foods gradually; don't try to make too many changes all at once.
- Above all, eat to live – don't live to eat.

THREE QUALITIES OF FOOD

	SATTVIC FOOD	RAJASIC FOOD	TAMASIC FOOD
Found in	• Pure, wholesome, naturally delicious ingredients	• Processed foods, salty and heavily spiced foods	• Stale or inedible foods, tasteless ingredients
Food types	• Fresh and dried fruits, berries and fruit juices • Raw, lightly cooked and steamed vegetables • Wholegrains • Legumes • Nuts and seeds • Fresh herbs, herb teas	• Onions, garlic • Refined sugar, soft drinks • Chocolate • Coffee, black tea, caffeinated beverages • Convenience foods and processed snacks • Also tobacco	• Meat, fish, eggs • Food that is overcooked, burned or barbequed • Fried food • Stale food • Items that are full of preservatives • Alcohol • Also recreational drugs
Effect	• Increases vitality, strength and endurance • Eliminates fatigue • Promotes cheerfulness and serenity • Boosts mental clarity • Helps maintain day-long mental poise and equilibrium	• Can over-stimulate body and mind • Associated with physical and mental stress • Not recommended for the circulatory and nervous systems	• Can lead to feelings of dullness • Associated with lack of motivation and purpose • May aggravate chronic ailments and depression

FASTING
To give your system a rest and promote healing

Most spiritual traditions recommend fasting as a purifying practice, often combined with vigil, as a means of strengthening prayer and meditation. In India, many people fast twice monthly, on the *Ekadasi* days (the eleventh day of each lunar fortnight).

Choosing to abstain from food for a short period – even a day – gives the digestive system a rest, allowing the body to cleanse itself thoroughly and making the energy that usually goes into digesting food available for repair and healing. The whole system is given an overhaul, and many people experience a resulting lightening of mind as well as body. Fasting also helps to develop concentration and willpower.

In the strictest sense, "fasting" means abstaining from all food, but this can be difficult without practice. At the beginning, you might like to sip juiced fruit with a good amount of water or take vegetable broths to stimulate the cleansing effect. It is important to drink as much water as possible while fasting to flush out your system, and herbal teas, especially peppermint, are helpful. Avoid black and green tea, coffee and fleshy fruit, such as bananas. Start by fasting one day a week, or miss one evening meal a week. Pick a time when you don't have to work and can be quiet. You may like to fast on your own, but sharing a fast with others can help reinforce your resolve.

Caution: Avoid fasting during pregnancy or breastfeeding, if you have diabetes, hypo-glycaemia, anaemia or an eating disorder (past or present). Consult a doctor or healthcare professional if you have questions or would like to fast for more than three days.

ONE-DAY FASTING
One day of fasting a week maintains good health and mental resolve, and it's easy return to a balanced diet next day. Or practise less often, as even an occasional fast is beneficial.

WEEKEND FASTING
Build up your stamina slowly with an occasional weekend fast. These are recommended several times a year, to rid you of stagnant energy.

EXTENDED FASTING

Just as you strengthen muscles with progressively more weights, so you can strengthen your mind with increasingly difficult challenges. Long fasts of a week and more are valued by more experienced practitioners for giving great spiritual strength and willpower. After Day 3, you may find your hunger disappears, but do break your fast safely (see below).

FASTING PRACTICE TIPS

- Try not to think about food; devote time instead to quiet activities.
- Ease headaches or nausea by drinking hot water with a little lemon or peppermint tea.
- Stay hydrated by drinking plenty of water.
- Do yoga poses; they will help eliminate toxins. Other light exercise, such as walking, is recommended but be careful not to tire yourself out.
- Practise breathing exercises to assist the detox process. Focus your attention on the cleansing out-breath, exhaling fully.
- Keep warm and rest as much as possible.
- Bathe frequently to relax your muscles and assist the skin's cleansing process.

SAFELY BREAKING A FAST

Resist the impulse to give in to cravings or heavy foods. Begin eating again slowly.

Day 1: Eat raw or stewed fruit to gently restarts the digestive system's peristaltic action.

Day 2: Add a raw vegetable salad meal to sweep out toxins accumulated in the intestines.

Day 3: In addition, eat lightly steamed vegetables. Avoid salt or seasonings – your cleansed palate will be able to better experience the natural flavours of food.

Day 4: Reintroduce grains to your diet. Or combine grains and vegetables in a meal.

Day 5: Return to a well balanced diet; try to avoid rajasic or tamasic food (see page 99).

CLEANSING THE LIVER
To rid your system of toxins

As the body's main detoxifying organ, the liver has more than 500 functions, including ridding the body of waste, metabolizing hormones and assisting in digestion. Boosting liver health to remove toxins is an integral part of any yoga cleansing programme.

Caution: Avoid with chronic stomach or digestive disorders or constipation, during pregnancy, menstruation, and with eating disorders (past or present). If you take medication or have questions, consult a doctor or healthcare professional.

SIMPLE DAILY DETOX DRINK

If you feel daunted by a full liver cleanse, support your liver and organs in eliminating everyday toxins by combining the following ingredients in a blender. Drink immediately.

150–200g (6–8oz) dark leafy greens, such as spinach or rocket

8g (2 tsp) chia seeds

1 lemon or ½ grapefruit, peeled

PREPARING FOR A 24-HOUR LIVER CLEANSE

The week before a cleanse avoid foods that tax the liver and eat more alkaline-forming foods, which are anti-inflammatory and help reduce stress levels in the body.

Avoid: fried and fatty foods, avocados, olives, nuts and seeds, salad dressing, dairy products, egg yolk, mayonnaise, cake, cookies, meat, alcohol, fizzy drinks.

Eat more: berries, citrus, melon, nectarines, pineapple, ripe bananas, figs, dates, raisins, asparagus, celery, kohlrabi, cabbage, broccoli, leafy greens, beans, endive, cucumber, root vegetables, mushrooms, tomatoes, wholewheat, alfalfa and barley grains, oregano, ginger.

Drink: fresh apple juice and eat apples: they contain pectin, a soluble fibre that binds to fatty substances in the digestive tract, facilitating their elimination.

EPSOM SALT CLEANSING MIXTURE

Make this up before starting the cleanse. Epsom salt is a natural mineral compound that acts as a detoxifying agent by increasing water in the intestines and replacing magnesium. Buy from a pharmacy or health store. You will also need 4 x 240ml (8oz) glass jars with lids.

60g (4 tbsp) Epsom salt (magnesium sulphate)
2 lemons (optional)

1 In each jar put 15ml (1 tbsp) of the Epsom salt and pour over 240ml (8oz) of water. Mix well, until the salt is dissolved. Squeeze 1/2 lemon into each jar to taste, if desired.
2 Put on the lids and store in the refrigerator until needed. Shake before using.

STARTING THE 24-HOUR CLEANSE

Choose a time when you can rest next day. Stop taking non-essential medicine, eat a no-fat breakfast and lunch, then avoid food and drink after 2pm. You will need:

4 servings of the Epsom salt cleansing mixture (see opposite)
1–2 grapefruit or 4–6 lemons or limes
125ml (4fl oz) organic extra-virgin olive or sesame oil (untoasted)
8–10 large apples, plus extra for juicing

DAY 1

6pm: Drink the first Epsom salt mixture. Then rinse your mouth with water, if desired.
8pm: Drink the next Epsom salt mixture.
9:45pm: Squeeze the grapefruit or lemons/limes into a large glass and add the oil. Mix thoroughly, but don't drink. Get ready for bed and visit the toilet. Take the third Epsom salt serving and the citrus-oil mix to bed.
10pm: Drink the citrus-oil mix over 5–15 minutes. Lie on your right side, knees pulled up to your chest. Try to sleep like this.

DAY 2

Early am: On waking, drink the third Epsom salt mix, then 600ml (1pt) warm water, if desired. Go back to bed.
2 hours later: Drink the final salt mix. Return to bed.
10am: Juice 5–6 apples and drink.
10:30am: Prepare a chopped apple salad or smoothie (skin on is fine). If you feel unwell, stick to apples and apple juice for the rest of the day.
Evening: Transition to light foods and salads.

CONCH-SHELL CLEANSE: SHANKH-PRAKSHALANA
To clear your digestive system

This cleansing treatment involves drinking saltwater while performing simple yoga exercises. The movements stimulate the water to cleanse your digestive tract, flushing out toxins, promoting healthy digestion and releasing stress. Because it is salty, the water is not evacuated as urine but reaches the colon and is absorbed there. The Sanskrit words *shankh-prakshalana* translate as "conch-shell cleansing" because the coils of the digestive system resemble the interior of a seashell. Yogis regard this as a natural way of cleansing the length of the alimentary canal. The cleanse is best done twice a year, with the changing seasons. Though it only takes 1–2 hours, rest and eat light food for the rest of the day.

Caution: Avoid with chronic stomach or digestive disorders, during pregnancy and menstruation, and with eating disorders (past or present).

PREPARING FOR THE CLEANSE
Choose a work-free day for the cleanse and eat lightly for three days before, avoiding meat, fish, eggs, dairy produce and alcohol. The night before the treatment eat a small meal, preferably of fruit. On the morning of the cleanse, mix 4–5 tsp sea salt into 4–5l (7–9pt) warm water (36–37°C or 96.8–98.6°F).

STARTING THE CLEANSE
- Drink 1–2 glasses of the saltwater then perform a round of exercises. Visit the toilet when needed. If you cannot get a desirable result massage your abdomen using clockwise strokes.
- Repeat the process of drinking saltwater, practising the exercises and visiting the toilet until clear water comes out of your colon. Then wait at least 30 minutes without drinking (or you will go to the toilet).
- Rest for the remainder of the day, drinking herbal tea or mineral water and eating kitchari – rice and lentils cooked together until soft, with a little added ghee (clarified butter) or sesame oil but no spices.

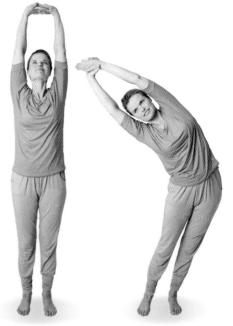

• For the next few days, avoid meat, fish, eggs, dairy produce and alcohol, but also raw fruit and vegetables, sour, fried and spicy foods, coffee, black tea and any foods that feel rich or heavy.

CLEANSING YOGA SEQUENCE

1 Mountain Pose (Tadasana): stand with feet approximately 30cm (12in) apart. Lift your arms overhead with elbows straight. Interlock your fingers and turn your palms up (see picture, top left). Give your body an exaggerated stretch; make yourself as tall as possible for 3–5 long breaths.

2 Crescent Moon Pose (Ardha-chandrasana): From Tadasana, bend as far left as you can. Do not twist; balance your weight between both feet (see picture, top right). Return to centre; bend to the right. Repeat 3–4 times to each side.

3 Standing Twist: Still in Tadasana, drop your arms. Gently swing them as you rapidly twist from side to side 3–5 times (see picture, right).

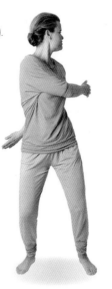

4 Cobra Pose (Bhujangasana): Lie on your abdomen, feet 30cm (12in) apart. Tuck your toes under and place your palms beneath your shoulders. Straighten your elbows to lift your body until only your palms and toes touch the ground. Turn to look over one shoulder as you twist your trunk, trying to see the opposite heel (see picture, bottom left). Return to centre; look over the other shoulder. Repeat 3–5 times on each side.

5 Spinal Twist (Ardha-matsyendrasana): Sit on the floor with legs out straight. Bend your right knee and place the foot flat on the floor outside your left thigh. Place your left hand on your right knee and twist as far to the right as possible, looking over your right shoulder (see picture, below right). Hold for 3–5 breaths then return to centre and straighten your leg. Bend your left leg and repeat to the other side.

CLEANSING THE UPPER DIGESTIVE TRACT: DHAUTI
To promote good digestive health

Everyday hygiene focuses on external cleanliness – bathing the body and brushing the teeth – but little thought is given to internal purification. The yoga tradition teaches that just as a machine needs regular servicing to ensure continued optimal functioning, so the human digestive system needs periodic internal cleansing to maintain good health.

Dhauti acts on the upper digestive tract – the throat, oesophagus and stomach – and encompasses a series of cleansing practices, from the simple swallowing of air to more complex procedures best practised with a teacher. Dhauti is one of the six classical yoga cleansing exercises or kriyas (see page 15) seen as the foundation for all other purifying techniques. It is said to help you pursue your life goals free from discomfort, fatigue and interruption. Even if you are not ready to try the method, it is worth understanding the principles.

Caution: Avoid dhauti during pregnancy and if you have an eating disorder (past or present).

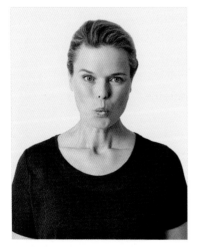

PURIFYING THE STOMACH WITH AIR: VATA-SARA

Commonly referred to as belching, this practice is said to eliminate the foul air that is a by-product of digesting "vata" (gas-forming) foods, such as beans and cabbage. It also counteracts the negative effects of eating too fast or not chewing food well.

1 Sit with your legs extended. Bend your knees to bring the soles of the feet together. Then place your hands on your hips.

2 Pull your cheeks in and try to bring your lips inward to create the shape of a bird's beak. Suck in air through your mouth and swallow it, trying to push the air down into your stomach.

3 When your stomach feels extended, try to contract it and push the air out.

PURIFYING THE STOMACH WITH WATER: VAMANA DHAUTI

Also known as *kunjal kriya* or *gaja-karani*, this advanced practice uses water to cleanse the stomach. For experienced practitioners, it is advised to practise once a week, first thing in the morning on an empty stomach. If using saltwater, before you start mix 4–5 tsp sea salt into 4–5l (7–9pt) warm water (36–37°C or 96.8–98.6°F).

At first practise under the guidance of an experienced teacher.

1 Drink at least 8 glasses of saltwater or regular water. Gently massage your stomach.
2 Using the index and middle fingers of one hand, tickle the root of your tongue until the water is vomited up.

PURIFYING THE STOMACH WITH CLOTH: VASTRA DHAUTI

This practice for more advanced yogis uses gauze to cleanse the upper digestive tract, and is valued for removing excess mucus, acid, gas and other impurities from the stomach. It is said to help asthma, heartburn, acid reflux, dyspepsia, indigestion, bloating and related problems. It may be practised once a fortnight or monthly on an empty stomach, preferably first thing in the morning. A roll of gauze 5cm (2in) wide, a bowl of slightly salted water, a larger empty bowl and some drinking water are required.

Always practise under the guidance of an experienced teacher.

1 Begin with a 1m (3ft) strip of gauze; increase it gradually until you are practicing with 5m (15ft).
2 Unroll the gauze into a glass of salty water.
3 Bring one end of the wet gauze onto one of your back molars. Begin to chew slowly to stimulate the swallow response. A little water helps wash the cloth down. To calm the gagging reflex, it's useful to stop for a moment and take a few deep breaths. This is not a hurried procedure.
4 Leave at least 5cm (2in) of gauze hanging from your mouth. The cloth can stay in for a few minutes while you practice Agni Sara or Nauli (see pages 108–109).
5 Give a gentle tug on the gauze; it will come up more quickly than it went down. Discard the gauze when you are finished.

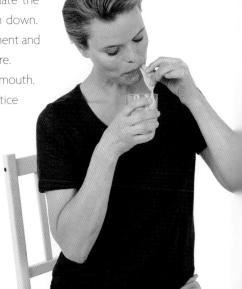

ABDOMINAL CHURNING: NAULI
To invigorate your whole system

Uddiyana Bandha and Agni Sara help you to control the abdominal muscles and are the first steps in mastering the important yoga cleansing practice of Nauli (see opposite), which stimulates the abdominal viscera and cleanses the entire gastrointestinal tract. Practise the exercises several times a day, or as often as you like, on an empty stomach.

Caution: Avoid nauli during pregnancy or menstruation, and if you have high blood pressure, heart problems, an ulcer or hernia.

HARNESSING UPWARD-MOVING ENERGY: UDDIYANA BANDHA
A static version of Nauli, this is a powerful exercise in its own right. Uddiyana Bandha stimulates the abdominal region and lungs, inspiring peristalsis and improving the function of the entire digestive, respiratory and eliminatory systems. It is particularly effective after Neti (see page 74) to activate Udana, your transformative "upward-moving energy" that governs the growth of your body, your ability to stand and speak, and your enthusiasm. Harnessing this positive energy helps develop your body and evolve your consciousness.

1 Stand with your feet a little more than hip-width apart and knees slightly bent. Lean forward at the waist and place your hands on your thighs, keeping your elbows straight.
2 Inhale deeply. Now exhale strongly through your mouth, emptying the lungs completely.
3 Keeping your breath out, lower your chin into the clavicle notch at your breastbone, tuck your tailbone under and try to pull your diaphragm upward. Feel as if there is a string at the back of the throat lifting the diaphragm. Simultaneously, pull your navel up and back. Hold for as long as you feel comfortable, with the breath out.
4 Release the upward-pulling action and allow your in-breath to come in naturally. Return to normal breathing, then repeat 3–5 times.

CLEANSING WITH INNER FIRE: AGNI-SARA
The Sanskrit term *agni-sara* means "fire essence". This initially challenging exercise vigorously contracts and expands the abdomen, giving the internal organs the exercise they need to function at optimal level. It stimulates digestive "fire" by invigorating the liver, spleen, stomach, intestines and pancreas. Regular practice is valued for relieving constipation and reducing abdominal fat. Practise on an empty stomach, preferably first thing in the morning.

1 Begin with Uddiyana Bandha, standing (as above) or sitting cross-legged. This lifts your diaphragm into the thoracic cavity freeing you to manipulate the abdominal muscles.

2 With your breath out and diaphragm in a raised position, contract and relax your abdominal muscles quickly. Repeat the vigorous pumping until you need to inhale, then release Uddiyana Bandha, let the in-breath come naturally and return to normal breathing.

3 Begin with 1–2 rounds, pumping 15–20 times in each round. Build up to 3–5 rounds daily.

ABDOMINAL CHURNING: NAULI

This advanced technique – pulling the diaphragm up into the thoracic cavity while exercising the abdominal muscles separately – is one of the six key cleansing processes or kriyas of hatha yoga (see page 15) and is said to use the inner "fire" of the body to regenerate and invigorate. Nauli is quite difficult and best learned from an experienced practitioner. Practise several times per day, or as often as you like, on an empty stomach.

1 Begin with Uddiyana Bandha while standing (see opposite). Keeping your breath out and diaphragm raised, contract the muscles on the left and right sides of the abdomen, bringing the abdominals into a vertical central line: Madhyama Nauli (middle contraction) (see picture, below left).

2 Keeping your breath out and diaphragm raised, contract the muscles on the left side of your abdomen, pressing your left hand into your left thigh and bending your trunk slightly forward to the left (Vamana Nauli) (see picture, below middle). Do the opposite on the right side (Dakshina Nauli).

3 Finally try churning: keeping your breath out and diaphragm raised in Uddiyana Bandha, rotate the abdominal muscles in quick succession from central nauli to the left and right (see picture, bottom right). When you need to inhale, release the abdominal muscles and breathe normally.

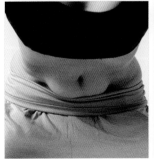 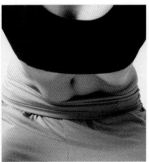 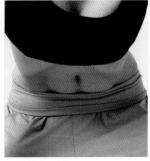

CLEANSING THE LOWER DIGESTIVE TRACT: BASTI
To reset your system

There are various methods of cleansing the lower digestive tract, including colonic irrigation, and using an enema bag. All these methods are recommended to help eliminate digestive problems associated with the three Ayurvedic constitutions (see pages 20–21) – whether your digestion is troubled by excess gas (an imbalance of vata), mucus (kapha) or acidity (pitta). More generally, cleansing the colon relieves blockages throughout the digestive system to leave you glowing with vibrant energy.

A more advanced technique is Basti, valued by yoga practitioners as a natural way of cleansing the colon with water, and one of the six key cleansing processes or kriyas of hatha yoga (see page 15). Even if you are not ready to try the method, it is worth understanding the principles. Basti is recommended to relieve chronic constipation, sciatica and lower back pain.

Caution: Avoid Basti during pregnancy or menstruation and if you have high blood pressure, diabetes, a hernia, polyps, colon cancer, diverticulitis or rectal bleeding.

COLONIC IRRIGATION

This hydrotherapy technique flushes the system of unwanted matter. An experienced therapist uses a machine to introduce warm filtered water into your colon through a small tube called a speculum that is gently inserted 4cm (1.5in) into the rectum. The water pressure and temperature are carefully controlled and waste is drained away discreetly in a closed system with no mess or smell.

This filling and emptying is repeated several times as the therapist gently massages the abdomen. Colonic hydrotherapy reaches the entire length of the large intestine, with the massage from the therapist helping to ensure an effective cleanse.

GRAVITY-CLEANSING THE COLON (ENEMA)

A gravity feed, more commonly known as an enema, can be used to cleanse the colon and stimulate peristalsis in the large intestine. In place of water, some people like to use very dilute herbal teas, such as peppermint, liquorice or ashwagandha, an Ayurvediic herb. Alternatively, 1–3 drops of essential oil (peppermint, frankincense or lavender) may be added to the water to encourage peristalsis and boost immune function. This is best practised in a comfortable place with space to lie down and within reach of a toilet.

1 Fill an enema bag or jar with warm water 36–39°C (98–103°F) and hang or stand it at least 60cm (2ft) above your body. Use a non-petroleum lubricant (olive or sesame oil or hand cream) on the enema tube.

2 Lie on your back or right side. Insert the lubricated tube into the colon and allow the water to start flowing. Keep the regulator at hand to control the flow of water. If there is any cramping, stop the flow of water immediately and take a few relaxing breaths. When you are ready, take a big breath and open the water valve again to resume filling the colon. Continue until 1–3 litres (2–5 pints) of water has been taken in.

3 Gently massaging your abdomen can assist the flow of water into the entire colon, but only take in as much as is comfortable. Then remove the tube and release the water into the toilet. This process may be repeated several times.

PERFORMING BASTI

Unlike colonics or enemas, which cleanse the rectum and the bottom 20–25cm (8–10in) of the colon, the more difficult Basti is valued for strengthening the muscles of the colon. Traditionally Basti is practised while squatting in water, and water is drawn into the colon as the muscles are contracted. A small (10–20cm/ 4–8in) bamboo or plastic tube may be inserted into the anus to aid the process.

Avoid Basti during pregnancy or menstruation and if you have high blood pressure, diabetes, a hernia, polyps, colon cancer, diverticulitis or rectal bleeding.

Although the original texts call for this technique to be practised in Chair Pose (Utkatasana), Garland Pose (Malasana) (see below) is easier. However, if you are not used to squatting, you may also find this pose rather difficult at first.

1 The yogi stands in a body of water or half-filled bathtub with feet slightly wider than hip-width apart, toes turned out at a 45-degree angle, then sits between the feet, as far down as possible. It's alright for the heels to lift a little. The elbows come inside the knees and the palms press together. This is Malasana. If a tube is being inserted into the rectum to help with drawing up the water, this is when it is done.

2 Still in the pose, the anal sphincter is contracted and relaxed as the yogi focuses on drawing water up into the colon. The water is held in the body for as long as is comfortable, then (removing the tube if inserted) the water is released into a toilet.

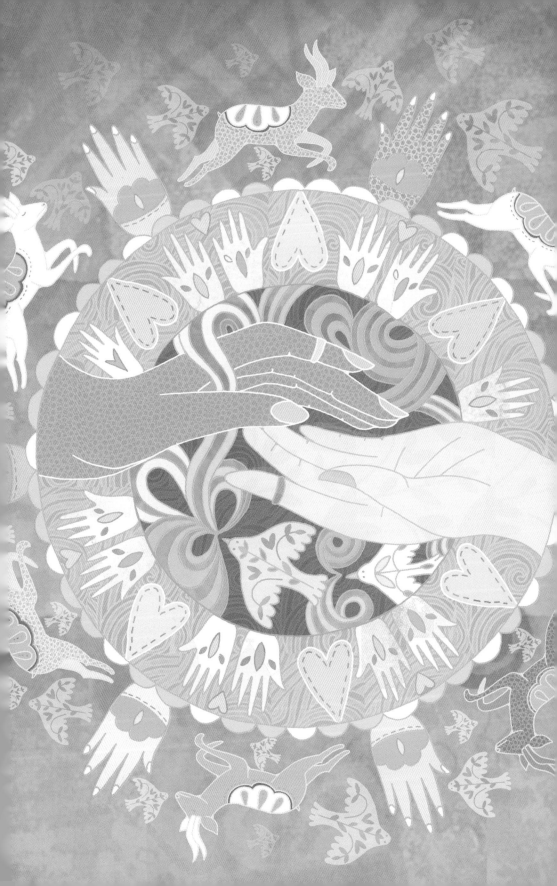

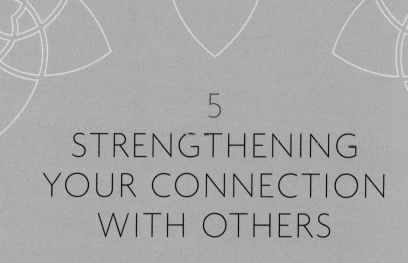

5
STRENGTHENING
YOUR CONNECTION
WITH OTHERS

TO LET GO OF TOXICITY AND LET IN FRESH AIR

*"Have a heart that never hardens and a temper that
never tires, and a touch that never hurts."*
Charles Dickens, *Hard Times*

*"Fire entered into the mouth taking the form of the organ of speech; Air
entered into the nostrils assuming the form of the sense of smell; the Sun
entered into the eyes as the sense of sight; the Directions entered into the
ears by becoming the sense of hearing; the Herbs and Trees entered into the
skin in the form of hair (the sense of touch)."*
Aitareya Upanishad, I–ii–4

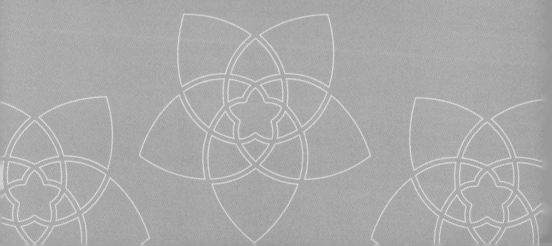

SENSITIZING YOUR SKIN – FOR TOUCH WITH COMPASSION

If you have a yoga practice, you'll know that one of its joys is a feeling of lightness and freedom. Skin-cleansing techniques enhance this experience. Your body's largest organ of elimination, skin offers extraordinary potential for detoxification. Cleansing programmes speed up the natural processes by which cellular waste is shed to allow new tissue to form, and sweat glands release toxins as they cool the body. Cleansing also enhances the ways in which life touches you and you interact with the world, skin being your intermediary.

THE SENSE OF TOUCH IN YOGA

Your skin contains a fine network of neural receptors that form your body's largest sensory system and enable you to perceive the size, shape, structure and texture of the world around you. These tactile points are responsible for every sensation you feel: cold, hot, smooth, rough, pressure, tickle, itch, pain, vibrations and more. Yoga philosophy relates your sense of touch to the element air or wind; it is the physical sensation your skin receives in its role as mediator between your inner and external environments.

EFFECTS OF CLEANSING THE SKIN

Skin has several layers. The one you see, the epidermis, is composed of dead cells that slough off constantly. A waterproof protective wrap for underlying layers and everything inside your body, it performs best if treated to daily baths or showers (see pages 120–21) and clothed in natural fibres that allow it to "breathe". Drinking plenty of water also helps the skin to perform its functions (see page 119). The epidermis contains sensitive touch receptors that feed the brain information about your environment. Deep-cleansed skin makes you more sensitive to such stimuli, for greater connection to the world around you. Smooth, soft hands also maintain sensitivity, which decreases with age. After cleansing, apply moisturizers containing vitamin E and organic shea butter, jojoba or avocado oils.

The second layer of skin, the dermis, contains sweat and oil glands, blood vessels and nerve endings. Its main function is to support the epidermis. New cells form at the junction between the dermis and epidermis, slowly pushing their way toward the surface. Sweat glands eliminate waste more effectively when pores are open. Saunas and steaming (see pages 116–17) and daily skin brushing (see page 118) promote this while increasing lymphatic flow to remove toxins and stimulating nourishing bloodflow. Exposing skin to short periods of sun is a good addition to a daily cleansing routine, stimulating production of vitamin D, which protects against osteoporosis, weak nails, fatigue and depression. Move into the shade after half the time it takes your skin to burn or apply sunscreen that blocks UVA and UVB light. There is a mantra to invoke the purifying light of the sun on page 131.

TOUCH AND YOUR ENERGY BODY

In yoga philosophy, touch is seen as a manifestation of the air element, matter in gaseous form. One of the easiest ways to purify your environment is to let fresh air into your home. Try a daily air bath by spending at least 10 minutes near an open window. You might even enjoy a "dew bath" by rolling on wet grass in the early morning.

Air is the element of the heart (anahata) chakra and expansive by nature (see page 19). When the heart chakra is purified and open you are able to give of yourself, express love unselfishly and be compassionate. Then it is possible to accept whatever life has to offer. The loving-kindness meditation on page 129 helps cleanse this chakra, while the throat and thoracic cleansing exercises on pages 126–27 free the region of physical and emotional tension. Working with the energy of the heart chakra helps you find emotional balance by aiding the release of stress, grief and other pent-up emotions (see page 128).

THE POWER TO CONNECT

Your skin and heart chakra are where life "touches" you, and cleansing your heart chakra enhances your ability to form and maintain loving partnerships. This chakra controls minor chakras in your hands that help you "reach out" to others. To enhance this, try the hand-chakra cleansing on page 124 and practise the many mudra hand gestures in the chapter, including Shaucha Mudra to rid you of tension and stimulate prana flow (see pages 122–23), and Apana Mudra to boost the natural expulsion of waste (see page 125). You will find a purifying ritual to help you connect all aspects of life, spiritual and physical, on page 130.

BENEFITS OF CLEANSING YOUR SENSE OF TOUCH

• Removes dead skin and pushes toxins out of cells.
• Stimulates your immune system by optimizing blood and lymph circulation.
• Inspires positive thinking and helps you maintain an optimistic outlook on life.

SAUNAS AND STEAMING: SVEDHANA
To promote healthy energy flow

Steaming and sweating therapies effectively dislodge and liquefy toxins in the body, and are widely used in Ayurveda, India's traditional medical system, to stimulate the flow of impurities from tissues into the digestive system, from where they can easily be expelled. Svedhana forms part of the Ayurvedic deep-cleanse treatment known as Pancha Karma (see page 22). Heat increases circulation to the surface of the skin, improves digestion, reduces muscle stiffness, and promotes restful sleep, while inducing sweating benefits cardiovascular health and is deeply cleansing for the skin. Time in a sauna or steam room can leave you feeling refreshed, relaxed, radiant and ready for whatever life has to offer.

Caution: Avoid if you have high blood pressure and during pregnancy and menstruation. Steam can exacerbate asthma and arthritis; consult a healthcare professional.

USING A SAUNA

Saunas provide dry heat and are usually hotter than a steam room, suiting those who like to sweat. Showering beforehand promotes sweating, enhancing the benefits. Saunas are good for arthritis and osteoporosis exacerbated by damp because dry heat can reduce pain, swelling and stiff joints, enhancing mobility and quality of life.

1 Wait 2 hours after eating. Drink lots of water; shower to promote sweating if desired.

2 Sit in the sauna for no more than 10 minutes, sipping water as required.

3 Take a cool shower then return to the sauna for another session, if desired.

4 Wait at least 2 hours before eating, though juice or a little fruit are fine.

USING A STEAM ROOM

The damp heat of steam rooms is more hydrating for skin and hair than dry saunas. Pancha Karma treatments often use a steam cabinet to keep the head cool as the body sweats. this can be replicated by wrapping your head in a cool wet towel in a steam room. If planning an enema, colonic or Basti (see page 110), a steam-room session can enhance its efficiency, but drink lots of water. Steam times recommended in the Ayurvedic tradition vary according to your constitution (vata, pitta or kapha):

Vata constitution: You tend to be fast-moving, thin and fine boned with a 'dry' body – a short steam time is recommended, 5–10 minutes.

Pitta constitution: Your fiery personality and oily skin indicate that you are "hot" already – choose the lower temperature of a steam room over a sauna session, 5–10 minutes.

Kapha constitution: You tend to have a solid body frame and calm temperament – you can withstand the highest temperatures and longest sessions, 10–15 minutes.

THE CLEANSING POWER OF HONEY

After sitting in a steam room for a few minutes, it can be nice to rub 15–30ml (1–2tbsp) of organic honey into your skin and continue steaming for a while more – then take a shower. Honey is antibacterial and hydrating and its antioxidants help repair the skin.

MAKING A FACIAL SAUNA

To unclog pores and leave skin glowing with health try a facial steam. It softens dead cells on the skin's surface and stimulates, encouraging new cell production. It also cleanses nasal passages in preparation for Nasya (see page 84). You will need a large bowl and towel. For dry or mature skin, add 250ml (8floz) milk to the water.

1 Fill the bowl with boiling water. Tie hair back, place a towel over your head and lean 25–30cm (10–12in) over the bowl. Close your eyes and breathe deeply through your nose for 5–10 minutes, or until the steaming stops.

2 Pat your face dry, tone – try the Morning Herbal Eye Wash (see page 38) and moisturize.

RESPIRATORY STEAMS

Follow the facial sauna instructions above but add any of the ingredients below to the water (the amounts below are per every litre (1.75pt), then breathe through your mouth.. This promotes deep and easy breathing and alleviates cold and sinus symptoms by releasing excess mucus from the linings of the throat, sinuses and lungs.

Caution: Essential oils should be avoided if you are pregnant or breastfeeding.

1 clove garlic, peeled and crushed

3–4 bay leaves, crushed

1–2cm (½in) slice of fresh ginger root, crushed

10–12 cardamom seeds, crushed

5–15ml (1–3tsp) fresh peppermint leaves

3–5 drops essential oil of eucalyptus, lemon or oregano

DRY BRUSHING
To boost vitality

Brushing skin with a stiff dry brush removes the uppermost layer of dry dead cells known as "scurf", a coating that holds onto acidity and toxins. This exfoliation, known as dry brushing, allows your skin to "breathe" and creates a new surface that can more readily eliminate toxins. Brushing skin also promotes movement within the lymphatic system and increases blood circulation and the healthy flow of the subtle energy yogis call prana. Brush your skin first thing in the morning, before eating.

Skin brushing has some of the benefits of exercise, enhancing circulation of blood and lymph, and enhances most yoga practice. It leaves you feeling more alert, refreshed and awake, and is helpful if you are trying to reduce your caffeine intake. The positive effects of skin brushing are enhanced if you drink water afterward.

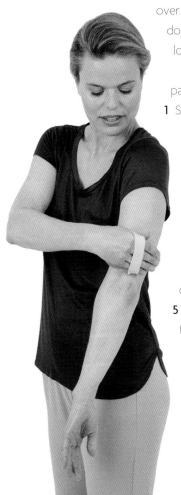

You will need a moderately stiff brush, preferably with natural-fibres. And if you prefer a handle, a long one makes it relatively easy to reach all over the body. Reserve this brush for skin brushing only, and don't allow it to get wet, which can cause the bristles to lose their effectiveness. Always brush towards your heart.

Be careful not to dry brush over varicose veins, painful rashes and open wounds.

1 Start brushing on the top of the right foot. Brush upward using gentle but brisk strokes. Work your way up your whole right leg and hip.

2 Repeat on the left foot, working up to the hip as before.

3 Then brush up from your right hand to your right shoulder. Repeat on your left arm, working up to the shoulder using brisk but gentle strokes.

4 Brush the front of your torso from the neck downward, always stroking toward the heart.

5 Repeat on your back, working down from the neck as far as you can reach, again stroking toward the heart.

6 Finish by gently brushing over your abdominal area, making clockwise strokes with the brush.

DRINKING WATER YOGA PRACTICE
To flush your system

Drinking a good quantity of water first thing in the morning enhances any cleansing programme and can ease or reduce the frequency of many health symptoms, from headaches to the pain of arthritis, and digestive disorders such as gastritis, diarrhoea and constipation. But drinking water and then practising this yoga sequence is even more beneficial as it encourages circulation to the abdominal region, helps removes blockages in the intestines and stimulates the urinary system to eliminate toxins more efficiently.

Practise early in the morning, using heated or room-temperature water. You may need to urinate a little more after practising.

Caution: Avoid if you are pregnant or menstruating

1 First thing in the morning drink 2–4 glasses (600ml–1l or 1–1.75pt) water. Build up gradually from 1 glass, adding the juice of ½ lemon, if desired.

2 Immediately kneel with your buttocks on your heels. Make each of your hands into soft fists with the thumb inside your gently clenched fingers. Place the fists on either side of your navel, thumb end upward (see picture, top right).

3 Inhale deeply. As you exhale, bend forward, bringing your forehead to rest on the ground. Do not lift your buttocks away from your heels (see picture, right). Hold for 5–10 breaths, breathing through both nostrils.

4 Sit up slowly. Wait at least 45 minutes before eating or drinking.

VARIATION: TO EASE TIGHTNESS

This relieves tension in the neck, upper back and shoulder muscles and improves circulation in the upper body.

1 Kneeling with your buttocks on your heels, clasp your hands together behind your back.

2 Straightening your elbows, lift your arms as you bring your forehead to the ground, then continue as for the main sequence (see picture, right).

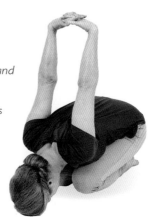

DETOXIFYING BATHS
To encourage relaxation

Classical yoga traditions advocate bathing before beginning physical poses (asana), breathing (pranayama) or meditation in order to prepare you for the internal cleanse of the practice. Then wait at least 30 minutes after bathing. The *Hatha Yoga Pradipika* advocates rubbing any perspiration into your body to make it "firm and light". You might like to add the following ingredients to bathing water, alone or in combination.

Caution: Avoid baths if you have high blood pressure, and during pregnancy and menstruation.

Epsom salt (magnesium sulphate): Through osmosis, magnesium is absorbed into your body, inducing calmness. Simultaneously, sulphates flush out toxins, easing stiffness, headaches, migraines or joint inflammation. Add 250g (9oz) to a full bath.

Baking soda (sodium bicarbonate): Increases the alkalinity of your body, leaving you feeling refreshed and with silky skin. Add a handful to a bath.

Colloidal oatmeal: Finely ground oats help absorb excess oil, prevent pores from clogging and relieve the discomfort of itchy dry skin, which often has a high pH level. Oatmeal's anti-inflammatory properties also help reduce swelling, redness and irritation. Add 250g (9oz) to a bath. Colloidal oatmeal can make the bath slippery, so bathe with care.

DETOX BATH RECIPE

Combine the following in a bowl and then empty into your tub under the running water as the bath is filling. Relax in a comfortably warm bath for 10–20 minutes.

50g (2oz) each fine sea salt, Epsom salt, baking soda (150g or 6oz in total)

75ml (3floz) apple cider vinegar

10 drops in total of one or a mix of essential oils (optional):

Bergamot: Regulates cravings, lifts spirits.

Grapefruit: Decreases mucus during detoxification.

Lavender: Nerve tonic for headaches, anxiety, depression and stress.

Lemon: Stimulates immunity and brings clarity to mind and emotions.

Peppermint: Cleanses the lymphatic system and stimulates sluggish digestion.

Oregano: Anti-viral and antioxidant.

Juniper: Supports elimination and liver function.

CLEANSING HOT AND COLD WATER
To promote circulation

Alternating hot and cold showers or baths creates a healthy flow within the circulatory system, which in turn stimulates the lymphatic system. It removes sub-cutaneous water retention, or "bloat", enhancing your ability to do yoga poses and sit for longer in meditation. In the yoga tradition this practice is considered particularly beneficial if you tend to procrastinate, experience frequent sore throats or find your work is hindered by stagnant energy.

When the body is warmed, a greater volume of blood moves to the surface (the skin). This promotes movement within the lymphatic system, enhancing elimination. Heat also increases pitta in the body, valued by yogis for removing excess cholesterol. With this dissolved, toxins can more easily leave cells and enter the lymphatic system for removal.

When the body is cooled, blood moves from the extremities toward the core. The body uses latent heat from deep within to warm itself. Alternating heat and cold increases the movement of both blood and lymph, leading to increased elimination.

ALTERNATING HOT AND COLD SHOWERS
This cleansing treatment works at any time of day, but it is especially useful first thing in the morning to help the body start moving after the stagnation of lying asleep overnight.
1 Begin by taking a normal warm shower.
2 Gradually turn the temperature to cool; stay in the water until your body feels cold.
3 Turn the gauge back to hot and remain under the shower until your body feels warm. Repeat the process 2–3 times, ending with a cold shower.

HOT AND COLD TUBBING
This is more extreme than showering as you stay in for longer. It should be avoided if you have a heart condition or high blood pressure. If you are pregnant, consult a doctor or healthcare professional before practising.
1 Lie in a warm bath with a cold wet towel on your head to prevent overheating.
2 Gradually add hot water until you reach your comfort limit. Relax for up to 20 minutes.
3 Run in cold water until you begin to feel cold. Get out of the bath and dry off. Put on warm clothes, including socks and a hat if desired, and go to bed with a hot water bottle.

DETOX GESTURE: SHAUCHA MUDRA
To reconnect with your inner essence

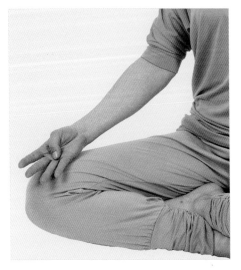

Practising the hand gesture known as Shaucha Mudra supports and intensifies the effects of a detoxifying diet and the practice of kriya cleansing routines (see page 15), which are further enhanced when you fast regularly (see pages 100–101). Pressing your thumb into the base of your ring finger has the energetic effect of decreasing the heavy and debilitating effects of stagnation within the body.

The gesture is said to stimulate the subtle energy known as prana to flow with the vigour and freshness of an unobstructed river. It is valued for systematically aiding the elimination of the accumulated tensions, toxins and negative emotions that tend to hinder good circulation on all levels. This includes the physical circulation of blood and oxygen, as well as the more subtle movements of energy and healthy ideas.

Shaucha Mudra can be practised with one or both hands and you may hold it while lying down, standing (such as while waiting for a bus), walking or sitting – even while watching TV. Bring the tip of your thumb to touch the base of your ring finger and press down gently – there is no need to push hard. Allow the hand and fingers to remain relaxed as you sustain the pressure with the thumb for up to 15 minutes daily.

CLEANSING VISUALIZATION
Shaucha Mudra is most effective when combined with the healing visualization that follows. If you fast regularly, or are planning to fast, this mudra and visualization practice assists the process and makes the cleansing experience more effective and healing.

1 Sit in a comfortable meditation position with your spine straight and head erect (see pages 24–25); do not lie down. Ground zyourself by breathing into the parts of your body that are in contact with the ground: your buttocks, legs and feet. Feel as though you are growing energetic "roots" deep into the earth. Every time you inhale, visualize yourself drawing up positive energy from the earth. With each exhalation, let go of a little of any impurities or negative emotions you may be holding on to.

2 After 10–12 deep breaths leave your "roots" in the earth and bring your awareness to your forehead. If you prefer, bring one hand about 5cm (2in) in front of your forehead, palm facing your head. Place the other hand 5cm (2in) in front of your heart centre, at the middle of your breastbone (see picture, below left).

3 Visualize a silver tube connecting your brow (ajna) chakra, also known as your "third eye" (see page 19) with your heart (anahata) chakra. Picture yourself inhaling through your forehead and visualize the air travelling down through the tube to your heart centre, and exhale from your heart centre. Then breathe in through your heart and out through the third eye.

4 Continue this process of breathing in through the third eye and out through the heart, and reversing to breathe in through the heart and out through the third eye.

5 After 2–3 breaths, drop your hands and allow them to rest on your thighs in Shaucha Mudra (see pictures, opposite and below right). Try to hold for at least 10–15 minutes, visualizing all blockages between these two important chakras dissolving.

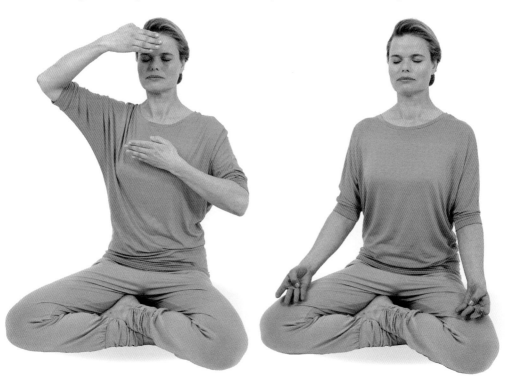

STRENGTHENING YOUR CONNECTION WITH OTHERS

PURIFYING THE HAND CHAKRAS
To sensitize your palms

The palms of your hands contain minor chakras that act as antennae, equipping you to receive and transmit energetic information. The sequence below cleanses and sensitizes your palms to bring you into contact with your own energy fields. Activating your hand chakras makes you more sensitive to therapeutic energy, the first stage in developing the ability to scan auras. The exercise also allows you to experience the direct connection of energy centres in your hands with your heart (anahata) chakra (see page 19).

1 Sit or stand, extending both arms in front of you, parallel to the ground, elbows straight. Turn your arms so one palm faces up and the other down.

2 Make fists and release them quickly, opening and closing your hands 20–30 times (see picture, below left).

3 Reverse the direction of your hands, turning the upward-facing palm down and vice versa. Repeat the rapid opening and closing hand movements 20–30 times.

4 Open your hands and turn the palms to face each other (see picture, below right). Slowly bring them together. When 20–30cm (8–12in) apart, you may feel a subtle ball of energy between your palms. Move them away from each other and back again. Play with the energy, bouncing it from hand to hand.

5 Now hold one hand 10–15cm (4–6in) in front of your breastbone, palm facing your body. Close your eyes and slowly begin to move your hand in a clockwise movement. After a few minutes reverse the direction, moving your hand anti-clockwise. Do you sense the movement of prana and have an experience of your heart chakra?

INCREASING SENSITIVITY
Rub 1 drop of essential oil of rose (to channel loving energy) or lavender (to increase sensitivity to other people's vibrations) into your palms to clear and activate your hand chakras.

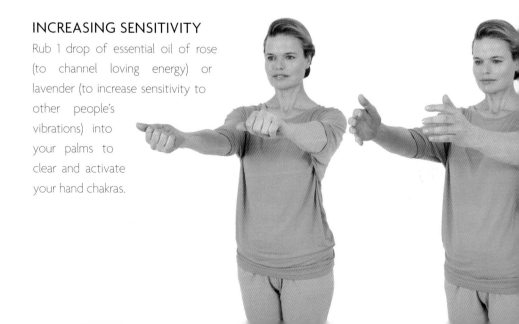

CLEANSING GESTURE:
APANA MUDRA
To boost immunity

The Sanskrit name for the cleansing aspect of the subtle energy yogis refer to as prana is *apana*, which means "moving outward". Apana governs all forms of bodily elimination: sweat, stool and urine; the expelling of semen, menstrual fluid and the foetus in childbirth; and the elimination of carbon dioxide through your out-breath. On a more subtle level, this cleansing energy purges you of negative sensory, emotional and mental experiences.

Apana supports healthy immune function on all levels, and Ayurveda, the holistic traditional medicine of India, regards the erratic movement of apana as the cause of many illnesses, including high blood pressure, heart palpitations, heart attacks, disorders of the respiratory tract and even schizophrenia.

You can practise Apana Mudra at any time and it is considered especially beneficial for women, helping to regulate the menstrual cycle and easing childbirth. It may be performed with one or both hands while you are sitting, standing or lying down.

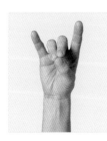

APANA MUDRA

Bring the tips of your middle and ring fingers to the top of your thumb. Allow your other fingers to remain extended and relaxed. Hold for up to 45 minutes daily.

Holding Apana Mudra while in a lying position known as Corpse Pose (Savasana) can have a particularly cleansing effect.

1 Lie on your back with your legs at least 60cm (2ft) apart. Let your arms rest away from your sides, both hands in Apana Mudra with palms facing up.

2 Close your eyes and gently seal your lips. Allow the breath to move rhythmically in and out of your nostrils; be aware of the sound of your breath moving in and out.

3 As you inhale, hear the breath say the word "let". As you exhale, hear it repeat the word "go". Do not strain or force your breath, just listen to the words "let" and 'go' with each in-breath and out-breath. Visualize yourself letting go of a little physical and emotional strain with each exhalation. Practise for 5–10 minutes.

CLEANSING THE ANAHATA CHAKRA: HRID DHAUTI
To release physical impurities

The heart (anahata) chakra controls our sense of touch. It is also the energy centre related to self-acceptance, compassion, forgiveness, trust, hope and emotional self-empowerment (see page 19). Purifying the heart chakra enhances your ability to reach out and touch others – and to allow yourself to be touched by the joys of life. Although the Sanskrit word *hrid* literally means "heart", most Hrid Dhauti practices, including the ones below, focus on cleansing the back of the throat and oesophagus. This stimulates a release of physical and emotional impurities from the thoracic region and heart chakra.

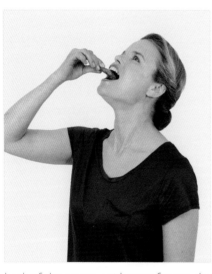

THROAT CLEANSING

Traditionally, turmeric root is used in the practice that follows, but a wooden tongue depressor may be substituted. Turmeric has a warm, bitter taste and is a strong antioxidant with antiseptic and anti-inflammatory properties. Try to buy the longest piece of turmeric root available, then steam to soften. When cool, apply a little ghee (clarified butter) or (untoasted) sesame oil.

Aim to practise first thing in the morning, on an empty stomach. If you don't have turmeric or a stick, simply massage the back of the tongue with your fingers, though this is not as effective.

1 Standing near a sink, take a deep breath as you lift your chin and tilt your head back slightly. Open your mouth wide and gently massage the back of your tongue with the turmeric stem or wooden stick (keep a good grip on it).

2 When you need to release your breath, or if you gag, stop and remove the root or stick. Take a few breaths and repeat. This massage stimulates the release of mucus, acidity and general impurities from the oesophagus; spit them out.

3 Repeat 2–3 times if desired. Then rinse your mouth with water.

THORACIC CLEANSING

This form of Hrid Dhauti practice cleanses the heart chakra at the energetic centre of your subtle body and helps to connect your physical and spiritual realms of being. The physical pose stretches the thoracic cavity, chest, hips and neck, and is said to be effective if you have backache and sciatic pain or urinary disorders. If you find the exercise too tricky, try Lion's Yawn Pose (Simhasana, page 56), which has similar benefits.

Caution: If you are new to this thoracic cleansing, it is best to practise with an experienced teacher.

1 Balance on your knees with your big toes together and your knees wide apart. Place your hands flat on the ground in front of you and walk them forward, keeping your elbows straight. Arch your spine downward and drop your pelvis as close to the ground as possible, without bending your elbows.

2 Then, open your mouth and eyes wide and exhale fully, sticking out your tongue. Hold the breath out, trying to look as ferocious as possible (see picture, below).

3 When you are ready, inhale fully as you relax your tongue, drop your head and allow your hips to move back toward your feet. Hold the breath in for as long as comfortable.

4 Repeat 3–5 times, moving your upper body backward and forward as you hold the inhalation and exhalations.

> "By steady focus on the heart chakra,
> a full understanding of the nature
> of the mind is gained".
> Patanjali's *Yoga Sutra*, 3.34

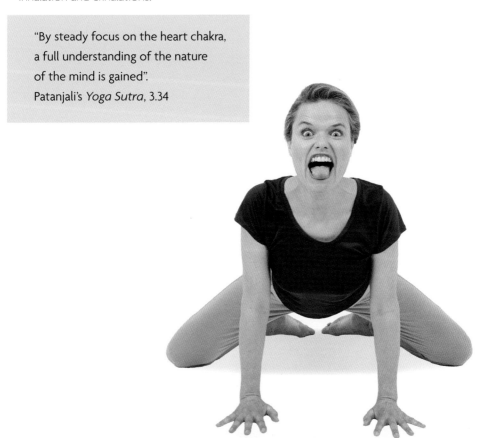

ANAHATA CHAKRA MEDITATIONS
To help you let go and forgive

Purifying the heart chakra with these meditations can help you release pent-up emotions, unburden your heart and get in touch with others on a deeper level. Long-lasting healing – of your body and relationships – usually involves a deep cleansing of the heart chakra.

LETTING GO OF GRIEF MEDITATION

Grief is the emotion of loss; when life has touched you in a negative or painful way there may be a feeling of emptiness in the chest cavity. The hurt and sorrow stem from your attachment: even though someone has physically gone, you are having trouble letting go of your attachment to them. But the more you hold on to the sorrow, the longer healing will take. This meditation encourages you to do the kindest thing, and move on.

1 Light some candles in a warm quiet room. Sit in a comfortable meditation position with your spine straight and head erect (see pages 24–25).

2 Recall a situation in which you felt a sense of wellbeing and contentment. Breathe deeply as you take a few moments to mentally re-establish that happy scene.

3 Now let go of the details of this scene, but continue to pay attention to the feelings of wellbeing. You may experience a warmth or glowing feeling in your chest region.

4 Visualize your heart as an unopened flower – perhaps a rose. As you focus on the bud, see it slowly beginning to open; feel your heart opening too. Notice a healing warmth radiating out from your heart and instilling a sense of wellbeing throughout your body.

5 Repeat this visualization several times if you prefer. Return to it when you feel particularly tense or are dwelling on grief or loss of any kind.

COMPASSIONATE HEART GESTURE: HRIDAYA MUDRA

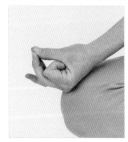 When you sit for meditation, bend the index finger of each hand until the tip touches its own base; keep rolling the finger down until the first knuckle touches the base of your thumb. Join the tip of the thumb and tips of your ring and middle fingers. Let the little fingers remain extended but relaxed and rest your hands on their respective thighs, palms facing up, as you meditate.

LOVING-KINDNESS MEDITATION

Doing a Loving-Kindness Meditation can help you to let go of stress and negativity while enhancing your ability to form and maintain loving heart-centred relationships. On a physical level, it is valued in the yoga tradition for easing stress related problems, including high blood pressure. On an energetic level, it offers a powerful cleanse of the heart (anahata) chakra as it allows you to override any negative feelings or thoughts you have either towards yourself, friends or family, or even people you feel have injured you. With regular practice, this can free you from much emotional suffering.

1 Sit in a comfortable meditation position with your spine straight and head erect (see pages 24–25). Bring your hands into Hridaya Mudra (see opposite). Close your eyes and bring your awareness to the centre of your chest. Take a few deep breaths and then let your breath find its natural rhythm.

2 Begin with self-healing by mentally repeating the phrases: "May I be happy. May I be healthy. May I live with ease. May I be free of dis-ease."

3 When you feel ready, move on to picture the face of someone you care about; maybe a friend or family member. Feel their presence, then direct the phrases of loving kindness to them: "May (name) be happy. May ... be healthy. May ... live with ease. May ... be free of dis-ease."

4 Next call to mind someone you don't know as well who is going through a difficult period. Imagine the warmth of your heart radiating out to this person. Mentally repeat the same words: "May ... be happy. May ... be healthy." and so on.

5 Finally think of someone who has injured you in some way. Forgive them. Feel your heart communicating compassion to that person. Mentally repeat the phrases again.

6 As your heart chakra opens, memories of past grief may come to mind. Be easy and nurturing with yourself. You may find it helpful to end your meditation by repeating the mantra "May all beings everywhere be happy and free.", or in Sanskrit *Lokah samasta sukhino bhavantu.*

> "Before you speak, let your words pass through three gates:
> At the first gate, ask yourself, 'Is it true?'
> At the second gate ask, 'Is it necessary?'
> At the third gate ask, 'Is it kind?'"
> Rumi

PURIFYING RITUAL: ACHAMANA
To prepare you for yoga practice

Doing the below traditional Hindu cleansing ritual before practising yoga can boost the efficacy of your practice. Its main functions are to awaken vital powers that drive away lethargy and cultivate gratitude for your physical, mental and emotional faculties. As you touch each body part in this ritual, visualize the gesture removing impurities. You will need a glass of water and small spoon.

1 Sit in a meditation position (see pages 24–25) with the water and spoon. Pour a spoonful of water onto your hands; mime washing them. Pour a small amount into your right palm and drink from the base of the hand. Repeat 3 times. Mime washing your hands again.

2 Put a few drops of water into your right hand. Place your right hand over the left without touching, and then move them along as though wiping your hands, then reverse the hands and do the same again (see picture, below left).

3 Using the bottom of your right palm, mime wiping the lower lip from right to left – then the upper lip from right to left.

4 With your right hand make a motion of sprinkling water, first over your head (see picture, below middle), then over your left hand, then your feet.

5 Make a loose fist with your right hand and place it beneath your chin.

6 Join the tips of your index finger and thumb of your right hand: use them to touch your right nostril and left nostril (see picture, below right).

7 Still using your right hand, bring the tips of your ring finger and thumb together and touch your right eye and then your left eye; your right earlobe and then your left earlobe.

8 Bring the tips of your little finger and thumb together and touch your navel.

9 Press the palm of your right hand flat on your breastbone, the heart chakra location.

10 Take your joined fingers to touch the top of your head.

11 Bring the tips of your thumb and middle finger together and touch your right shoulder and left shoulder.

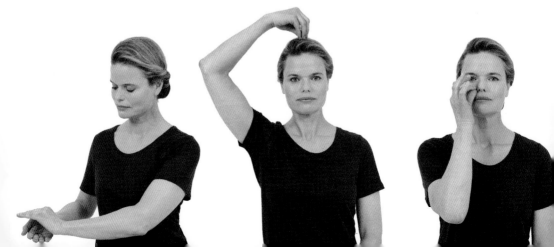

PRANAYAMA WITH GAYATRI MANTRA
To purify with sound

In this breathing practice, best performed first thing in the morning, you repeat a variation of one of the best known Sanskrit mantras, Gayatri, which invokes a light that can purify every part of your being. The mantra, which is explained further in the chart below, is a hymn to Savitur, the sun, offering gratitude both to the physical sun and the divine light that shines in all beings.

Don't worry if you struggle saying any of the words, the cleansing power of this exercise lies in the process itself rather than in perfect pronunciation.

1 Sit in a comfortable meditation position (see pages 24–25). Inhale for 5 seconds.

2 Place your hands in Vishnu Mudra, closing your right nostril with your thumb and your left nostril with your ring and little fingers (see page 78).

3. If comfortable, hold your breath for 20 seconds while you repeat Gayatri mantra:
"OM bhur,
OM bhuvaha,
OM Suvaha,
OM Mahaha,
OM Janaha,
OM Tapaha,
OM Satyam,
Om Tat Savitur varenyam bhargo devasya dhimahi dhiyo yona prachodayat,
OM apo-jyotir-rasomritam Brahma Bhur Bhuva Suvarom".

4 Then remove your fingers and exhale for 10 seconds. Repeat this 5–10 times.

Repeat during breathe retention	Refers to cleansing of
Om bhur	Physical body, experienced when you are awake
Om bhuvaha	Subtle/mental body, experienced during dreaming
Om Suvaha	Causal body, containing the karma
Om Mahaha	Consciousness of the liberated state
Om Janaha	Body of knowledge
Om Tapaha	Body of light
Om (nasal) Satyam	Body of truth
Om Tat Savitur varenyam bhargo devasya dhimahi dhiyo yona prachodayat	The ultimate inner light
Om apo-jyotir-rasomritam Brahma Bhur Bhuva Suvarom	May I experience that pure consciousness beyond all bodies

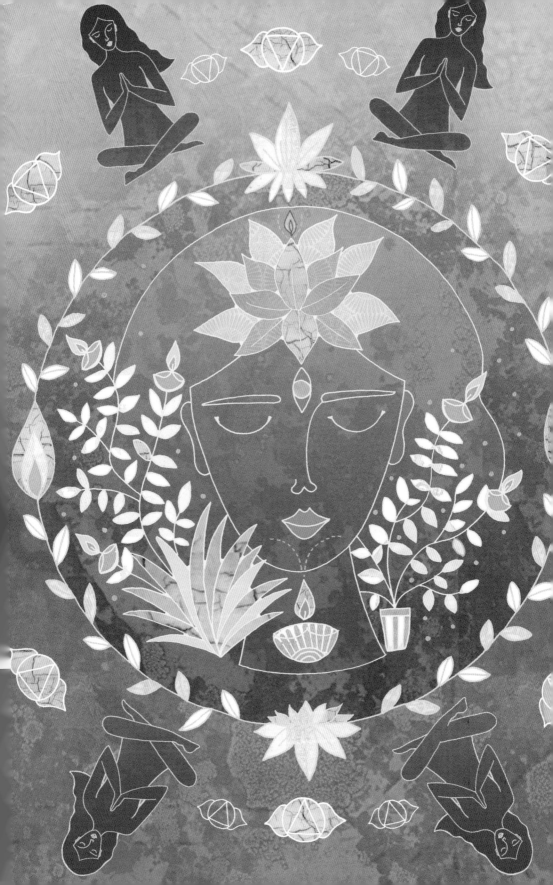

6
SIMPLIFYING
YOUR LIFE

TO DECLUTTER AND MAKE SPACE FOR HAPPINESS

"We are shaped by our thoughts; we become what we think.
When the mind is pure, joy follows like a shadow that never leaves."
The Buddha

"Yoga is the peace you experience when your mind is absolutely calm."
Patanjali's *Yoga Sutra*, 1.2

CLEARING YOUR MIND – TO FILL WITH SUBLIME THOUGHTS

As the faculty that controls all the senses, the mind is called upon throughout yoga cleansing practices for its role in stilling thought, sensation and desire – all the possibilities that tug at your consciousness and disrupt your inner peace (see page 23). When the mind becomes more firm and strong as you engage in the purifying practices in this chapter, you may notice that you have increased self-control, feel less distracted by the sensory world and are more aware of your inner self, which is peaceful, vibrant and content.

THE MIND IN YOGA

Many people confuse the brain with the mind. The brain is in your physical body, but your mind is more subtle, existing in what yogis refer to as the "astral body" (see pages 16–17). Perhaps the best definition of your mind is a bundle of thoughts. If you could get rid of all your thoughts, your mind would theoretically cease to exist. However your mind is a living thing that wants to stay alive – and will strongly resist extinction.

Some meditation teachers suggest you try to "empty" your mind. But, if you were to sit and think, "I must empty my mind", your mind would be full of that thought rather than being empty. So instead, most teachers in the yoga tradition suggest that you try to focus your mind on one positive thought. In Patanjali's classic eight-part yoga system (see pages 10–11), concentration (*dharana*) is the step before meditation (*dhyana*).

Your mind is much more powerful than you realize, and when it is scattered you waste energy, making it difficult to realize your true potential. Yoga cleansing techniques let you uncover the vastness of your mind, which lies like an iceberg of hidden promise.

EFFECTS OF CLEANSING THE MIND

When you purify your mind and develop the ability to concentrate, your thoughts become very powerful. As an analogy, think about holding a magnifying glass over a piece of paper in bright sunlight. If the lens is clean, it focuses the sun's rays, perhaps strongly enough to set the paper alight. In a similar way keeping a journal of your thoughts and feelings, including negative self-talk that might be disempowering you (see pages 140–41, channels and magnifies your flow of consciousness by not allowing the flow to dissipate. In yoga philosophy, the mind (*chitta*) is likened to a lake upon which waves rise and fall.

These waves are your thoughts, *vrittis* in Sanskrit. A better definition might be a mental whirlpool – in the average mind thousands of vrittis arise in the mind every second.

When a lake is calm, with the waves stilled, you can see the bottom clearly. Likewise, when the vrittis of your mind subside you experience great inner peace. Yoga is the restraining of all mental activity, the calming of the fluctuations of your mind. In addition to being a series of techniques to control your thought-waves, the term yoga is also used to refer to the joyous state in which you experience deep peace.

THE MIND AND YOUR ENERGY BODY

The brow (ajna) chakra, sometimes referred to as the third eye, is the command centre of your subtle body (see page 19). It is the inner instrument whose job it is to manage your five senses (sight, hearing, smell, taste and touch) plus your mind – and to regulate all the other chakras.

CLEAN YOUR SPACE TO CLEAR YOUR MIND

Yoga teaches that happiness comes when you no longer rely on outside sources for joy in life. This chapter contains visualization techniques for detoxing some of the negative emotions that arise when we do – such as impatience, greed and anger – to restore contentment and balance (see pages 138–39). There are also decluttering tips to promote the art of simple living, ridding yourself of things that do not contribute to your ultimate happiness (see pages 142–43). You will find ways to create a greener space and cleaner air with purifying plants (see pages 146–47) and a ceremony for energetically purifying your environment with light and by burning incense and smudging herbs (see pages 144–45).

The mind is also purified when you act selflessly – then any ego and negative feelings begin to be replaced by tolerance and compassion, and you gain an awareness of the interconnection of all things. As your motives for acting become more purified by practising Karma Yoga (see pages 148–49), your mind becomes quiet and truly still.

BENEFITS OF CLEANSING YOUR MIND AND SIMPLIFYING LIFE

• Enhances perception in general.
• Helps you let go of disempowering thoughts and stimulates a positive attitude to life.
• Encourages you to declutter both your inner and outer environment.
• Strengthens your ability to channel latent capacities of mind.

CLEANSING AJNA CHAKRA
Purifying your mind's eye

The brow (ajna) chakra located at the third eye just above and between your eyebrows is the seat of your wisdom (see page 19). Purifying it can help you to reconnect with your inner wisdom – so you think more clearly, see the "big picture" in life, improve your memory, develop your imagination, connect with intuitional abilities, expand your consciousness and develop greater spiritual awareness. If impurities gather here, they may lead to feelings of confusion, uncertainty and inertia, and a cynical or pessimistic outlook. These cleansing techniques can clarify your thought processes and create a more harmonious balance between the various faculties of your mind. Practise anywhere and at anytime, especially if you feel depleted of energy.

1 Sit in a comfortable meditation position with your spine straight and head erect (see pages 24–25). Visualize your shoulderblades sliding toward your waist. This helps to keep your breastbone lifted and ensures the movement of your ribcage is unimpeded.

2 Close your eyes. Rub your hands together vigorously until you feel warmth generated between them. Gently cup your palms over your eyes and bathe them in complete darkness. Take 5–8 slow, steady breaths in and out before dropping your hands.

3 Bring your hands into Jnana Mudra by joining the tips of your index fingers with their respective thumbs, then rest your inner wrists on your thighs, palms facing down.

4 Bring your awareness to the centre of your forehead and inhale deeply through your nose. Keeping your eyes closed, draw in as much air as possible. Imagine you are drawing in much more than air; feel yourself also drawing in the subtle energy yogis call prana.

5 When your lungs are full, hold your breath for as long as is comfortable, visualizing the energy you have inhaled forming a sphere of bright light at the centre of your forehead. Use your mind's eye to see it as a vibrant ball of indigo light. If you watch it with full concentration, you might notice it giving off sparks – or even flashes of lightning.

6 When you are ready, exhale, watching the light dissolve into a warm, sparkling shower of energy. Repeat 5–10 times daily.

PURIFYING POWDERS

In Hindu tradition, three "powders" are traditionally applied to the third-eye area to purify the brow (ajna) chakra and enhance meditation and other yoga practices.

Vibhuti or holy ash: Represents Siva, the destructive aspect of the divine consciousness.

This grey powder helps dispel negative qualities.

Chandana: Represents Vishnu, the aspect of the divine consciousness that keeps the universe in balance. Sandalwood powder is mixed with water to form a cooling paste. Applied to the forehead, it balances the flow of energy at the brow (ajna) chakra.

Kumkum: Represents the goddess or Divine Mother, the creative aspect of the universe. A red powder made from flowers, this is used to stimulate and open the brow (ajna)chakra.

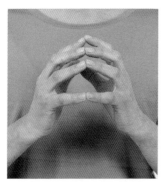

PROBLEM-SOLVING GESTURE: HAKINI MUDRA

Named for Hakini Shakti, the feminine dynamic force that personifies the energy of ajna chakra, this hand gesture improves and deepens respiration for a cleansing effect. It recharges the brain, enhancing memory and intellectual capacity by stimulating communication between the right and left hemispheres, and is recommended when you have intensive abstract work or mental puzzles to solve. You might try it when you have "lost the thread" of a conversation or need to tap into your intuition for guidance. It can be practised any time and any place.

1 Sit comfortably upright – this doesn't need to be a meditation position, but don't cross your legs or ankles. If possible, sit facing east.

2 Bring the tip of each finger to the tip of the respective finger on your other hand: for example bring the tips of each thumb to touch. Your eyes can be open or closed, but direct them upward, toward the centre of your forehead.

3 Take 5–10 deep breaths in and out. With each inhalation, bring the tip of your tongue onto the hard ridge just behind your upper front teeth. As you exhale, let your tongue relax. Notice whether your mind's eye begins to resolve your problems.

VARIATION: FOR LONGER CONCENTRATION

After taking the initial 5–10 deep breaths, continue to sit in deep contemplation with both hands in the mudra. Keep your eyes turned toward the centre of your forehead and maintain the synchronized movement of your tongue with your breath – this keeps you from drifting off. This variation may also help if you are seeking inspiration.

DETOXING NEGATIVE EMOTIONS
To restore balance and contentment

Purifying visualization techniques are used in yoga to dissipate negative personality traits, transforming them into more positive qualities. In yoga terms, negative emotions such as guilt, anger, rage, bitterness and jealousy are thought to relate to imbalances in various chakras (see pages 18–19). Anger, for example, is considered an impurity related to an imbalance in the solar plexus (manipura) chakra. Although the following exercises diffuse anger, you may also use them to help clear any emotion that is troubling you. All stimulate a gradual emotional cleansing on conscious and sub-conscious levels, and practising them regularly can help rid you of feelings that, if not cleared out, can lead to a lack of joy in life.

EMOTION-RELEASE VISUALIZATION

One of the basic teachings of yoga — and many other spiritual traditions — is to acknowledge a negative emotion, but not identify with it, and then release it. Whenever negative emotions come into your mind, notice the emotion but try not to dwell on it. Instead, detach yourself from the feelings by visualizing them as bubbles that rise to the surface of your mind and then "pop". Yoga teaches that if you do not identify with thoughts, they cease to exist within your consciousness.

AFFIRMATIVE VISUALIZATION

This technique, known as *vairagya*, or detachment, teaches you how to substitute a positive for a negative emotion. Sit to practise for 15–20 minutes daily. With regular practice the positive images will become so strong in your mind that they begin to become your habitual reaction. Negative responses weaken until eventually even deep-seated undesirable qualities are cleared away. Repeat at different sittings with other adverse emotions — for example, replace impatience with tolerance or greed with moderation.

1 Sit in a comfortable meditation position with your spine straight and head erect (see pages 24–25). Relax your shoulders. Breathe gently through your nostrils as you remind yourself of a negative quality — notice yourself "indulging" in this bad habit. For example, if you tend to get angry when you miss a train, visualize yourself standing on the platform as the train doors close in your face. Notice your usual response, for example you might watch yourself becoming angry and frustrated.

2 Run through the experience several times, as though replaying a film. Each time you watch, pick up on new details, including how your solar plexus feels.

3 Now change the scenario. On this run-through, instead of getting stressed-out, visualize yourself taking a deep breath and reminding yourself that there is no need to get upset. See yourself expressing the opposite quality: staying calm and unperturbed. If any anger persists, visualize yourself breathing it out.

LETTING GO OF ANGER

If you are constantly aggravated, feel irritated or resentful about small things or are easily provoked to sarcasm, cynicism and disdain, try this exercise, which is valued by yogis for clearing anger and associated "burning" emotions. Practise this technique in silence – make sure the TV, phone and other devices are off and turn down any music. You may engage in simple manual tasks as you practise, such as gardening, chopping vegetables or walking – activities that can be done with little intellectual engagement. It helps to give your hands to the work and your mind to the visualization.

1 Begin by remembering a time when you felt irritated. For instance, when you were late for an appointment and someone grabbed the parking spot you wanted.

2 Ask yourself, "Why did I get angry?" If the answer is "Because someone took my parking place" you are confusing the trigger with the underlying cause of your emotional outburst. Be aware that the immediate stimulus for your anger is not the real reason behind it.

3 Now consider another example: you are sitting in a cafe and someone puts their hands over your eyes. You might feel frightened and angry until you turn around and recognize an old friend. Your perception of the situation quickly changes and you no longer feel angry. Be aware that when you feel angry it is not because of what others have done but caused by your evaluation of a situation.

4 When you next feel a twinge of anger or irritation, ask yourself "Why am I getting angry?" and ponder the cause within you rather than the external trigger. Remember that this process is not about stifling anger or simply willing yourself to calm down. It helps you to identify and start to transform the inner causes of anger.

5 As you practise, analyse and better understand your reactions over time, notice how you feel cleansed of various degrees of irritation.

PURIFYING YOUR SELF-IMAGE
To enrich your personal growth

You many abstain from drugs, alcohol and cigarettes, but you may be harming yourself in more insidious ways if you unconsciously indulge in negative thought patterns or make self-demeaning statements such as, "I'm no good at this" or "I'm useless". By releasing such disempowering thoughts you can cleanse your view of yourself and become more friendly, compassionate, joyous and balanced. In his classic guide to yoga, the *Yoga Sutra*, the ancient sage Patanjali introduces four types of positive, life-affirming thoughts, referred to as the *chitta prasadanam* (mind-calmers; see below); Buddhists call them the *brahmavihara* (divine vehicles). By applying these four attitudes to your daily life you purify the mind and make it more tranquil.

MIND-CALMING YOGA THINKING

1 Friendliness: Make friends with happiness – feel pleased when you encounter people who are working on and succeeding in their spiritual practice or life in general.

2 Compassion: Have empathy for those suffering, not steering their life on a positive path or going through difficult times.

3 Joy: Take delight in the presence of good people.

4 Balance: Don't let negativity disturb your equilibrium.

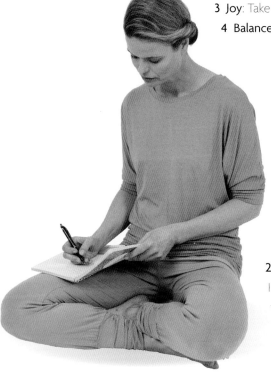

QUESTIONS TO ASK YOURSELF

To apply the four mind-calming thoughts observe your state of mind regularly by asking yourself these questions (or make up your own). Gradually you will find your thoughts becoming more concentrated and your mind more dominated by purity than by passion or inertia.

1 How friendly am I?

2 Am I compassionate toward people when I see them suffering? How benevolent am I toward my own failings?

3 Do I feel sincere joy when friends, colleagues and family are successful? How do I react when they succeed, but I fail?

4 Does my mind stay balanced when I'm with people acting ethically and morally wrong?

JOURNALING TO TRANSFORM HIDDEN THOUGHTS

When observing the mind, it's useful to be able to monitor changes in your attitudes towards the four principles of chitta prasadanam. That's easy if you record your findings in a dedicated journal. Begin by observing and recording your thoughts and reactions to the four questions. This stimulates positive change by bringing sub-conscious thoughts into your conscious mind. Connecting everyday feelings with deeper levels of consciousness helps you recognize connections and can change attitudes you weren't aware of.

1 Each morning (preferably after meditation), sit for at least 10 minutes and write whatever comes to mind – don't edit! You might use these questions to stimulate ideas:

- What are my strong points – how do I stop myself developing them?
- What negative attributes do I have? How real are they?
- Do I have self-doubt? How much do I allow it to control my life?
- Do I allow others to hurt me by not setting proper boundaries?
- In what ways am I afraid to succeed?
- Am I unnecessarily judgemental toward myself?
- Do I need the constant approval of others?
- How much do I rely on my inner resources?
- Am I a perfectionist who never seems to do things as well as I would like?

2 Write quickly; don't stop, noting down whatever comes to mind. You don't have to write full sentences; spelling and grammar don't count. No one will read what you write. Why not attach articles and images that relate to your inner purification in some way?

3 Write a dialogue with yourself, carrying on a conversation about the questions. You may not reach a conclusion, and don't be afraid to keep returning to key points.

4 While writing, become aware of the attitudes you have toward yourself and ways you may be harming yourself by putting yourself down, for example. Try not to be judgemental.

5 As your journal grows, regularly ask yourself "What can I do with this material?" "What is its deeper meaning?" This helps you begin to appreciate yourself, which enriches your personal growth and spiritual development.

CLEARING YOUR SPACE AND YOUR MIND
To simplify your life

Many yoga texts suggest that you can purify your life by cleansing your home of everything that is unnecessary and does not contribute to your ultimate happiness. The attitude is summed up in the words of yoga master Swami Sivananda, who advocated "Simple living and high thinking". When you live more simply, you cleanse yourself of the stressful distractions, temptations and expectations that can accompany an over-stretched lifestyle.

Start the process by taking time to reflect on what you regard as a "life necessity". Of course we all need the basics to live safely and healthily: a roof over our heads, somewhere to sleep, eat and work. But the yoga way is not to think of a bed, table and desk as objects that indicate success; rather they are instruments that assist you in accomplishing your goals in life. From a functional point of view, perhaps the only difference between a comfortable old desk and a brand new one is the belief that new is better.

Simplifying your life is not about giving up possessions. It is more about cleansing your mind of the belief that happiness depends on things outside yourself – this refers to relationships as much as material objects. The possessions-audit technique below will help you reflect on how far material possessions exert control over your life. Whether they influence the number of hours you work, for example, or the jobs you have to take on to earn enough to pay for everything. Then you can use the decluttering tips opposite to help you put this mind-cleansing to practical use in your home, offering easy ways to prevent the upkeep, protection and renewal of your possessions from controlling or overwhelming you.

POSSESSIONS AUDIT

Ask yourself these questions and you will begin to notice how attached or detached you are to your possessions. If you keep a journal, you might like to write your answers there, and return to them regularly. The answers might help you see how purifying your environment and living more simply could improve your life.

- Do I use "things" to reinforce my sense of identity?
- Do I resent having to share my things or space with others?

- Do I tend to hoard possessions I'll probably never use? How cluttered is my home with things I no longer need or love?
- Do I make things last or do I replace things quite often?
- Am I in the habit of judging people by the possessions they have collected?
- Do I surround myself with things that might enhance other people's opinion of me?
- What does it mean to need something?
- Do I tend to give or to take? How do I understand this phrase: "The true spirit of simple living involves deep generosity"?
- How might my joy in life improve if I lived in a simpler way?

DECLUTTERING TIPS

What do your home and workspace say about your state of mind? According to yoga philosophy, when your environment feels pure and light, you tend to be less encumbered by gross and subtle imbalances. So the condition of the space you inhabit has a direct connection to the quality of your health, wellbeing and inner peace. Clear one and the other tends to follow. Cleanliness and order lift self-esteem and reinforce your expectations that you are worthy of having good experiences. These tips can help you toward a more streamlined and clean home:

- Observe your state of mind in different surroundings and begin to notice which ones make you feel clear and transparent, and which do the opposite. Compare your mind when walking in a park or on a beach, for example, with standing on a crowded train or driving in congested traffic.
- Begin to declutter your living space by preparing a bag for the charity shop. Every day, put one item into the bag. When the bag is full, drop it off at the charity shop and prepare another bag.
- Make a resolve to straighten your desk, kitchen and workspace each day before you leave it.
- Clear out or reorganise at least one drawer or cupboard each week.
- Keep energy flowing smoothly within your environment by freeing it from piles of stuff – whether dirty dishes, laundry, unread magazines, unanswered mail or garbage.
- Notice your levels of focus and how easily you are distracted at a desk or worktop when it is clear and when it is messy.
- Clear a dedicated space in which to meditate or practice yoga postures – it is more motivating and easier to spend longer amounts of time in a place free from clutter.

PURIFYING SPACE
WITH LIGHT: ARATI
To make an environment more auspicious

You can purify your practice place morning and evening or at the end of any yoga or meditation session with the ritual of Arati. Whether a simple ceremony or extravagant ritual, it involves waving a light – burning camphor, an oil lamp or candle – around a space to energetically purify the environment. The light symbolizes spiritual knowledge and enlightenment, and is rotated clockwise, often on a plate, and accompanied by bells or singing. In India lights are waved and mantras chanted at the end of every meditation session, while thousands gather at pilgrimage places at sunset to wave lights and sing.

Purifying symbols and rituals like Arati can stimulate psychological cleansing. Camphor crystals burn with a pleasantly purifying scent and without leaving ash or residue. The philosophical analogy is drawn that when the ego is burnt through by the practice of yoga, only pure consciousness remains. The individual ego is visualized as melting like the camphor, with the *jivatman* (individual soul) uniting with the Supreme Light of Lights.

1 Hold the lamp in your right hand and rotate it clockwise around the space (see picture, below right). Picture it cleansing the room of residual negative energy. At the same time, visualize it cleansing your body and mind from inside and see yourself as that light moving out into the world.

2 Present the light to each participant, who will cup their palms over the flame and then symbolically touch their eyes, raise their hands to the forehead and then slide them down the body (see picture, below left).

3 Offer fruit or sweets to ensure the memory of the practice is sweet. In India no ritual or group practice is complete until food is shared.

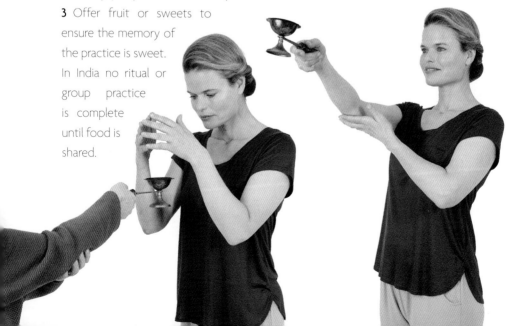

PURIFYING SPACE WITH INCENSE OR HERBS: SMUDGING
To clear unwanted energy

Burning incense and smudging with herbs or plant resins is used to physically and energetically purify an environment, clearing impurities, unwanted energies and negative emotions such as sadness, anxiety or dark thoughts that may be clinging to the space or to an individual. Incense is often burned during meditation and yoga practice; sandalwood, in particular is valued for its calming and centring effect on the mind. Smudging might be included in ceremonies or gatherings along with songs of purification and wellbeing. In Native American traditions smoke is regarded as a bridge to the higher realms, a way to attract good spirits while dispelling negative or stagnant energy.

You might choose to burn incense or herbs after an argument to "clear the air", when moving into a new home or to re-invigorate your current living space. Light the incense or herbs and fan smoke throughout the space or direct it over a person.

CLEANSING INCENSE AND HERBS
You cannot burn frankincense or myrrh directly, but need to place pieces of dried resin onto a burning tablet of charcoal.

Sandalwood: India's traditional incense. Clears and focuses the mind and helps to draw you into a meditative state.

Frankincense: Deepens and slows the breath as it sharpens, elevates and clarifies. Has a long history of use in cleansing, protection and to ease the transition into death.

Myrrh: Calms, brings tranquillity, and instils confidence, stability and a feeling of centring.

Cedar: Used to purify and drive out negative energy and usher in positive influences. Often burnt to bless a new home in Native American ceremonies.

Juniper: Used throughout history in purification rituals. Invigorates mind and body and helps reverse psychological stagnation.

Sage: The best-known ceremonial smudge plant for meditation, cleansing an environment and purifying individuals. Burn to remove energy left by a negative person or argument.

Sweetgrass: Once sage has removed negativity, sweetgrass can be burnt to attract positive energy into a space.

Mugwort: Subtly cleanses negative energy. Burn before bed to stimulate sweet dreams.

PURIFYING PLANTS
To tap into the cleansing power of nature

Clean air at home, work and in your yoga practice space is a prerequisite for health and wellbeing, and is associated with reduced stress and anxiety. It's best to choose a well-ventilated space for practising yoga and breathing exercises to guard against headaches, dizziness, nausea, and eye, ear and nose irritation. Reducing airborne pollutants such as mould is particularly important if you have asthma.

All plants absorb carbon dioxide and release oxygen, but some houseplants filter out airborne pollutants like dust, mould and household chemicals particularly effectively. The yoga tradition has long used plants as an environmental cleansing aid – neem trees are planted around Indian hospitals and ashrams (places of practice) for their ability to absorb large amounts of CO_2 (thanks to the large leaves and canopy), absorb pollutants and oxygenate the air. Mango, banana, coconut, sandalwood and banyan trees are also used.

THE CLEANSING POWER OF NEEM

Neem has been used for thousands of years for its antibacterial, antiviral and antifungal properties. The bark, leaves and seeds are valued in Ayurveda to relieve infections, promote clear breathing and treat diabetes. Traditionally twigs are used for brushing teeth.

SPACE CLEANSING WITH PLANTS

It seems that workers tend to be more productive when offices are filled with greenery, and hospital patients tolerate pain better in a ward containing plants. The most thorough investigation into the purifying effects of houseplants was conducted in the 1980s by NASA researchers, keen to maintain healthy conditions in space stations. Their Clean Air Study found that certain plants efficiently remove many chemicals linked to negative health effects. In the yoga tradition plants are seen to increase calmness and positivity as they clean the air. They can make a big difference in how you feel about your practice.

Garden chrysanthemum is the air-purifying champion, removing chemicals found in household detergents, paints, plastics and glue products.

Spider plants and most **cactuses** convert the positive ions from your computer into negative ones (see below). The spider leaves absorb mould and other allergens; it is the ideal plant if you have dust allergies.

English ivy is perfect for people with pets as it reduces the amount of airborne faecal matter. It is excellent for your yoga practice area as it reduces airborne mould.

Dracaena removes benzene found in dyes, formaldehyde in paints, trichloroethylene and xylene in solvents. Toxic to dogs and cats.

Peace lily absorbs mould spores through the leaves, circulating them to the roots as food.

Boston fern restores moisture to the air; perfect for dry skin and health problems exacerbated by cold weather.

Philodendron is best for homes without pets or children as the plant is toxic if eaten. However, it is an excellent choice for removing the formaldehyde found in particle board.

Bamboo palm is a superstar for filtering formaldehyde and benzene – partly because it can grow to 4m (13ft).

Aloe vera is an ideal bedroom plant, releasing oxygen continuously through the night. Also valued for its wound-healing, antibacterial and anti-inflammatory properties.

CLEARING POSITIVE IONS

An ion is an invisible charged particle in the air – a molecule or atom that has lost or gained an electron as a result of atmospheric forces or environmental influences. There are negative and positive ions; some research studies have linked exposure to negative ions to lower levels of stress, anxiety, depression and enhanced wellbeing. There are high concentrations of negative ions in the air of clean environments. This may help explain why we feel so empowered when walking near the ocean or running water.

Positive ions are produced by electronic equipment and air conditioning, and some people associate them with increased anxiety and irritability, tension or lack of energy felt, for example, when walking on a busy road or spending hours at a computer. Unfortunately, modern homes and workplaces have become chronic generators of positive ions. These particles are so small they can be absorbed directly into the bloodstream from the air we inhale, potentially affecting the lungs, respiratory tract and immune system.

Spider plants and cactuses convert potentially energy-draining positive ions to invigorating negative ions. So do Himalayan salt lamps, whose soft pink colour is the result of a high concentration of trace minerals. Water vapour in the air carries dust, pollen, dander, smoke particles and bacteria; the salt in the lamp attracts the water molecules and absorbs them along with the attached pollutants, meaning they are no longer airborne.

PURIFYING YOUR MOTIVES: KARMA YOGA
To move beyond yourself

Karma Yoga encourages you to perform actions because you think they are the right things to do, and to act without expecting a certain outcome or reward. This selflessness helps to purify your mind, removing any hint of negativity or selfish intentions.

The Sanskrit word *karma* signifies "action". It encompasses the thought of doing the action, the actual physical deed, and the result and repercussions of that action. In yoga philosophy the consequence of an action is not a separate thing, but a continuation of the action – part of an ongoing chain of action and reaction.

Contrary to what many people think, karma has little to do with fate, destiny or luck (good or bad). Instead it implies free will. Although you may not be able to change past events, you are free in the present to choose how you will react to their aftermath. If you want to change the direction of your life in the future, then you need to change your actions in the present.

Karma Yoga is the discipline of selfless action as a means of self-perfection; this selfless service brings a new and deeper meaning to life. As you practise, so egoism, hatred, jealousy and feelings of superiority begin to be cleansed from your mind – to be replaced by humility, selfless love, sympathy, tolerance and compassion. You start to acquire a broader outlook and a sense of the unity of all life.

Examples of Karma Yoga might include meditating with hospice patients, working at your local food bank, or offering your services to a charity without seeking remuneration. It's about using your energy to better the lives of others – and possibly society in general. The great Indian leader Mahatma Gandhi did not distinguish between menial service and dignified work – he regarded cleaning toilets as the highest form of yoga. Stories tell that when newcomers to his ashram felt shy about doing menial chores, Gandhi would do their work himself. Next day, people would willingly do the tasks assigned to them.

To replicate Gandhi's example, use every possible opportunity to serve others. Do it cheerfully and willingly, without expectation. In fact, thank the person who has given you the opportunity to serve! It is difficult to perform truly selfless service. There is often a niggling voice in your mind that wants to be thanked – or at least appreciated. But as your motives become purer, this noise will become quieter. The finest form of Karma Yoga is imparting wisdom. If you are generous with the knowledge you possess, your heart will expand more quickly and you will find the world is your home – there is no greater form of inner purification than spontaneous acts of Karma Yoga.

HOW TO BEGIN KARMA YOGA

- Consciously try to respect everyone and everything you encounter throughout the day, everyday.
- Do at least one "random act of kindness" daily – on your birthday, do at least five. Do them without thought of what you might gain or who might benefit as a result.
- Be generous with your time and resources. Lend an ear or a hand; give a gift or a compliment; support good causes in whatever way you can.
- When someone helps you in some way, "pay it forward" by doing something similar for another person.
- Become aware of your attitudes toward give and take in your relationships. Do you tend to always give or always take – or do you enjoy a healthy balance, as the situation requires? Work on developing deep generosity, preferably without making mental notes in your energetic account book.
- When you give to charity, give of yourself. Don't just give away things you don't want any more. Although there is nothing wrong with donating old clothes to charity, it doesn't help to open your heart or instil an attitude of loving-kindness and purity of motives.
- Although we say "it is better to give than receive", it is not possible to continuously give. It is also important to nurture yourself, through a regular routine of yoga postures, breathing, healthy diet and regular meditation. Karma Yoga requires that you keep your body and mind strong – if you are drained you will have nothing left to give.
- Look for Karma Yoga classes in yoga studios – the teacher donates their services and students make donations to support a charity or good cause.

"The mind is purified by cultivating friendliness towards those who are happy, expressing compassion towards those who are suffering, feelings of goodwill towards those who are virtuous, and not being disturbed by people whom we perceive as being negative or vicious".
Patanjali's *Yoga Sutra*, 1.33

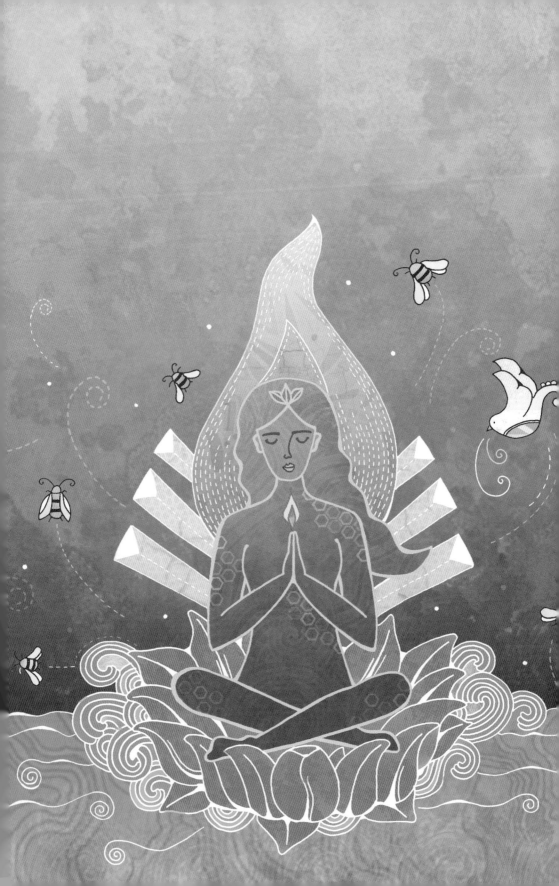

7
CLEANSING ROUTINES

PROGRAMMES TO BUILD OPTIMAL WELLBEING

In this chapter you will find daily, weekly and seasonal routines of cleansing exercises to help you maintain good health in body and mind. There are also suggested routines to ease the symptoms of common health conditions exacerbated by the stresses of modern life and by polluted water, air and food. The routines include general lifestyle advice alongside a range of techniques to suit your schedule and the amount of time you have to devote to cleansing.

For instructions on how to practise each of the recommended kriyas and cleansing techniques (and their specific benefits), turn to the page reference in the main chapters.

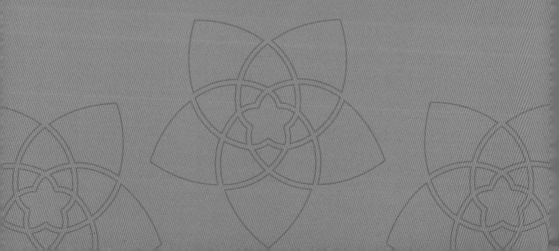

ROUTINES FOR GENERAL WELLBEING

Having a regular yoga practice and attending yoga classes, eating a healthy diet and cultivating a positive outlook on life encourages good health. But you can enhance these good habits and further develop your wellbeing by spending just 5–10 minutes a day weaving the cleansing exercises in this book into your schedule.

DAILY ROUTINE
• **On waking:** bathe your eyes (pages 38–39), clean your tongue (page 94), practise oil pulling (page 96), brush your teeth followed by gum massage (page 95) and dry brush your skin (page 118). Then do Neti (pages 74–75), Kapalabhati (pages 76–77), Alternate Nostril Breathing (pages 78–79) and sit in a meditation pose (pages 24–25) to practise one of the meditation and /or visualization exercises.
• **Anytime:** write in your journal (page 141) and do Karma Yoga (pages 148–49).

QUICK DAILY ROUTINE
If you have only a few minutes a day, try to include at least the following in your morning routine: Tongue Cleaning (page 94), tooth brushing (page 95), oil pulling (page 96), eye washing (page 38), Neti (page 74–75) and Kapalabhati (pages 76–77).

1 DAY A WEEK ROUTINE
• **Diet:** eat a light diet, low in proteins and carbohydrates and high in fresh fruit and raw or lightly cooked vegetables.
• **Meditation:** use the powerful cleansing meditative practice Tratak (pages 36–37) as your point of focus for 20–30 minutes at least once (unless contraindicated).

SEASONAL ROUTINE
• **Diet:** when winter becomes spring, and as summer is turning into autumn springclean your system with a longer fast of perhaps 3–7 days (pages 100–101).

ROUTINES FOR HEALTH CONDITIONS

All the exercises in the book are helpful to everyone (except when detailed in the cautions). But if you experience the following health conditions, it is helpful to add these extra cleansing exercises into your regular daily, weekly and seasonal routines for wellbeing.

STRESS, ANXIETY

Focus on the mind-cleansing exercises in Chapter 6 (pages 132–49), adding:

• **Daily:** neck exercises (pages 58–59), Ayurvedic face massage (pages 86–87), rejuvenating eye compresses (page 38), 1 hour of Mouna (page 61).

• **General advice:** spend time letting go of anger and other negative emotions; reduce your intake of coffee, tea, sugar and carbonated drinks (even sugar-free).

DEPLETED ENERGY, FATIGUE, EXHAUSTION

Try to rebuild a healthy flow of energy in your body to overcome feelings of stagnation and restore vigour by practising:

• **Morning:** dry brushing your skin (page 118) followed by alternating hot and cold showers (page 121), rejuvenating eye compresses (page 38), Nada-nu-sandhana (pages 62–63).

• **Evening:** chakra awareness meditation (page 48).

• **General advice:** reduce your intake of coffee, tea, sugar, chocolate (even dark), alcohol and carbonated drinks (even sugar-free).

INSOMNIA, SLEEP PROBLEMS

Focus on the mind-cleansing exercises in Chapter 6 (pages 132–49) to quieten your thoughts at the end of the day, adding:

• **Daily:** a yoga posture practice including Shoulderstand (page 57), and cleansing your chakras with light (page 49).

• **Evening:** before bed practise Chitra meridian visualization (page 45).

• **General advice:** eliminate coffee, black tea and energy drinks from your diet; limit your intake of chocolate (even dark) and sweets.

HEADACHES, MIGRAINES

Avoid Tratak (pages 36–37) and Drishti (page 46-47) with frequent migraines, and practise:
- **Preventative measures:** daily eye exercises, especially somatic movements (page 32–35), rejuvenating eye compresses and cleansing the third eye (pages 38–39), daily yoga posture practice including Tree and Banyan Tree, Dancing Siva and Eagle poses (pages 40–43).
- **Daily:** neck exercises (pages 58–59), cleansing your chakras with light (page 49).

DIGESTIVE PROBLEMS

Focus on the taste-cleansing exercises in Chapter 4 (pages 90–111), adding in:
- **Daily:** Uddiyana Bandha (page 108), Hrid Dhauti (pages 126–127).
- **General advice:** dine at midday, when digestive fire is strongest; chew thoroughly.

WEIGHT PROBLEMS

Focus on the taste-cleansing exercises in Chapter 4 (pages 90–111), adding in:
- **Daily:** alternate-nostril variation of Kapalabhati (pages 76–77), Eagle Pose (page 43), Shoulderstand (page 57).
- **Weekly:** fast for 1 day on water or fresh juice (pages 100–101); visit a sauna (page 116).
- **Seasonal:** Shank-prakshalana (pages 104–105).
- **General advice:** eat less and fewer rich, salty foods; have a regular yoga posture practice.

SKIN PROBLEMS

Focus on the touch-cleansing exercises in Chapter 5 (pages 112–131), especially:
- **Daily:** dry brushing your skin (page 118). Kapalabhati (pages 76–77)
- **Weekly:** visit a sauna (page 116).
- **Seasonal:** Shankh-prakshalana (pages 104–105).

ARTHRITIS, STIFF JOINTS

To remain mobile, focus on all the yoga postures in the book, adding in:
- **Daily:** practise Shaucha Mudra with the cleansing visualization for 15 minutes (page 122).
- **Weekly:** fast for 1/2 day, after lunch taking only water or fresh juice (pages 100–101).
- **Seasonal:** visit a sauna (page 116), liver cleanse (pages 102–103).

- **General advice:** eat a purifying diet (page 98–99), drink lots water and try to reduce your intake of coffee, tea and other acid-forming food and drink (see page 100).

ASTHMA

Focus on the scent-cleansing exercises in Chapter 3 (pages 70–89), adding in:
- **Daily:** Neti (pages 74–75), Kapalabhati (pages 76–77) and dry brushing your skin (page 118).
- **Weekly:** Nasya (pages 84–85), visit a sauna (page 116).
- **Seasonal:** beat pollen as spring turns to summer with respiratory cleanses (pages 70-89).
- **General advice:** eat a purifying diet (pages 98–99), try to reduce your intake of mucus-forming foods like dairy produce, and grains; eat lots of fresh fruit and green vegetables.

HAY FEVER, ALLERGIES

Focus on the scent-cleansing exercises in Chapter 3 (pages 70–89), adding in:
- **Daily:** Neti (pages 74–75) and Kapalabhati, including the alternate-nostril variation (pages 76–77), thoracic cleansing (page 127); Ujjayi as a breathing exercise (page 64).
- **Seasonal:** practise Neti (pages 74–75) 2–3 times a day during hay-fever season.
- **General advice:** try to reduce your intake of mucus-forming foods like dairy produce.

PREGNANCY

Many of the exercises in this book are contraindicated during pregnancy but will be of great help after childbirth. Drink plenty of water throughout your pregnancy, and practise:
- **Daily:** a yoga posture practice including Half Shoulderstand (page 57), chakra awareness meditation (page 48), Bhramari (pages 54–55) and at least 1 hour of Mouna (page 61).

AGEING

For a healthy posture and mental focus and to combat declining toxin elimination, practise:
- **Mornings:** eye exercises (pages 32–35), Tratak (pages 36–37), face massage (pages 86–87).
- **Daily:** yoga posture practice including Tree and Banyan Tree poses (pages 40–41), cleansing your chakras with light (page 49), 1 hour of Mouna (page 61).
- **Weekly:** visit a sauna or steamroom (pages 116–17).
- **Seasonal:** fasting (pages 100–101), liver cleanse (pages 102–103).

GLOSSARY

Ahamkara: ego; the sense of self as a separate entity

Ahimsa: non-violence in thought, word and action

Apana: the cleansing manifestation of prana

Aparigraha: non-greediness

Asana: seat; posture or position; yoga physical exercise

Asteya: non-stealing; non-covetousness

Ayurveda: traditional Indian medical system

Bandha: energetic lock

Brahmacharya: continence; control of sexual energy

Chakra: multi-dimensional ball of subtle energy; energy centre within the astral body

Dharana: concentration

Dhyana: meditation

Dosha: one of the basic constitutions of the body in Ayurveda

Ishwara-pranidhana: self-surrender or surrender of the ego

Kapha: mucus; water and earth dosha; one of the three basic constitutions in Ayurveda

Karma: action; results of action; the law of action and reaction

Kosha: sheath or layer

Kriya: cleansing action

Kundalini: dormant potential energy; primordial cosmic energy located in the individual

Mouna: voluntary silence

Mudra: energetic seal

Nadi: energy channel within the astral body

Niyama: internal discipline; ways to relate to yourself in a positive manner

Pitta: fire dosha; one of the three basic constitutions in Ayurveda; supplies the energy of catabolism that is essential for digestion

Prana: vital force; life energy; subtle energy that flows through the physical body

Pranayama: control or elongation of the prana

Pratyahara: withdrawal of the senses

Samadhi: enlightened or super-conscious state

Santosha: contentment

Satya: truthfulness

Shaucha (often written Saucha): purification

Swadhyaya: self-study; study of the nature of the self; study and chanting of spiritual texts

Tapas: austerity or voluntary simplicity; purifying action; production of inner heat

Vata: wind; air dosha; one of the three basic constitutions in Ayurveda

Yama: ethics, restraints; internal purification through moral training; positive ways to relate to others

RESOURCES

Swami Saradananda – may be contacted via her website: yogamentor.yoga
The Hatha Yoga Project – a research project based at SOAS, University of London, which aims to chart the history of physical yoga: https://www.soas.ac.uk/yoga-studies/

FURTHER READING

Classic texts on Hatha Yoga: *Hatha Yoga Pradipika, Gheranda Samhita, Shiva Samhita*

Cabot, Sandra, ***The Liver Cleansing Diet***, SCB International, 2012

Fife, Bruce N D, ***Oil Pulling Therapy***, Piccadilly Books, 2008

Frawley, Dr David, ***Neti: Healing Secrets of Yoga and Ayurveda***, Lotus Press, 2005

Jensen, Bernard, ***Tissue Cleansing through Bowel Management***, Book Publishing Company, 2011

Kingston, Karen, ***Clear your Clutter with Feng Shui***, Piatkus, 2008

Rajarshri Muni, Swami, ***Classical Hatha Yoga***, Life Mission Publications, 1997

Sadashivananda Tirtha, Swami, ***The Ayurveda Encyclopedia***, Ayurveda Holistic Center Press, 2012

Saradananda, Swami, ***Chakra Meditation***, Watkins Publishing, 2008

Saradananda, Swami, ***The Essential Guide to Chakras***, Watkins Publishing, 2011

Saradananda, Swami, ***Mudras for Modern Life***, Watkins Publishing, 2016

Saradananda, Swami, ***The Power of Breath***, Watkins Publishing, 2009

Satyananda Saraswati, Swami, ***A Systematic Course in the Ancient Tantric Techniques of Yoga and Kriya***, Bihar School of Yoga, 1981

Stevens, J C, ***Kriya Secrets Revealed***, Golden Swan Publishing, 2016

INDEX

ACKNOWLEDGEMENTS

Thanks to Dr Rajesh and Deepa Marattakalam of the Ayurananda Clinic in Pondicherry for both their care and their stimulating discussions; to our model Sarah Odell (Savitri) for her vibrant good health and inspiration; to Emma Brown (Radhika) for her "magical practise" and sharing of her knowledge of ayurveda. I'm planning to run retreats at Emma's Casa Santosha in Malaga, Spain - full information on my website: yogamentor.yoga. Undying gratitude to my teacher, Swami Vishnu-devananda, who not only guided me during his lifetime, but also gave me permission in perpetuity to quote from his works and teachings.